CORE CASES IN CRITICAL CARE

CORE CASES IN CRITICAL CARE

Edited by

Saxon Ridley
Consultant in Anaesthesia and Intensive Care
Norfolk and Norwich University Hospital
Norwich

Gary Smith
Consultant in Intensive Care Medicine and
Honorary Senior Lecturer in Critical Care
Queen Alexandra Hospital
Portsmouth

Anna Batchelor
Consultant in Anaesthesia and Intensive Care
Royal Victoria Infirmary
Newcastle

GMM

London • San Francisco

Typeset by Charon Tec Pvt. Ltd, Chennai, India

Printed in the UK by the Alden Group Ltd, Oxford

Distributed worldwide by Plymbridge Distributors Ltd and
in the USA by Jamco Distribution

Visit our website at **www.greenwich-medical.co.uk**

CONTENTS

PREFACE

This book describes the pathophysiology and clinical management of common problems seen in critically ill patients. Twenty illustrative case histories are presented and used as springboards to describe and discuss the principles that underpin successful treatment of the underlying conditions. Each chapter follows a standard format: definition or description of the problem, its pathology and pathophysiology, therapeutic goals, therapeutic options based on physiological or pharmacodynamic effects, usual outcome, key learning points and references for further reading. The chapter authors are all practising intensivists and the book reflects a consensus approach to the common clinical problems seen in both intensive and high-dependency care. The book is suitable for members of the multi-professional critical care delivery team, including trainees from anaesthesia, medicine and surgery, nurses and members of the allied health professions. It is, especially, relevant to trainees in these disciplines and to those revising for higher examinations. By providing a systematic discussion of common conditions, we hope to assist the reader in formulating their own case discussions.

Saxon Ridley
Gary Smith
Anna Batchelor

CONTRIBUTORS

Dr N. Barber FRCA, Specialist Registrar in Anaesthesia, Surgical and Anaesthetic Directorate, Queen Elizabeth Hospital, Gayton Road, Kings Lynn, NR 30 4ET, UK

Dr A. Batchelor FRCA, Consultant in Anaesthesia and Intensive Care, Royal Victoria Infirmary, Queen Victoria Road, Newcastle, NE1 4LP, UK.

Dr S.V. Baudouin MD, FRCP, Senior Lecturer in Critical Care Medicine, Department of Anaesthesia and Critical Care, Royal Victoria Infirmary, Newcastle upon Tyne, NE1 4LP, UK.

Dr M. Blunt FRCA, Consultant in Anaesthesia and Intensive Care, Surgical and Anaesthetic Directorate, Queen Elizabeth Hospital, Gayton Road, Kings Lynn, NR30 4ET, UK.

Dr S. Brett MD, FRCA, Consultant in Intensive Care Medicine and Anaesthesia, Department of Anaesthesia and Intensive Care, Hammersmith Hospital, Du Cane Road, London, W12 0HS, UK.

Dr A. Cohen FRCA, Consultant in Anaesthesia and Intensive Care, The Intensive Care Unit, St James's Hospital, Beckett Street, Leeds, LS9 7TF, UK.

Dr R. Craven MA, FRCA, Specialist Registrar in Anaesthesia, Frenchay Hospital, Bristol, BS16 1LE, UK.

Dr R.T.J. Cree FRCA, Specialist Registrar in Anaesthesia, Royal Victoria Infirmary, Newcastle upon Tyne, NE1 4LP, UK.

Dr G.P. Findlay FRCA, Consultant in Intensive Care Medicine, University Hospital of Wales, Heath Park, Cardiff, South Glamorgan, CF14 4XW, UK.

Dr C.S. Garrard FRCP, DPhil, Director, Intensive Care Unit, John Radcliffe Hospital, Headley Way, Headington, Oxfordshire, OX3 9DU, UK.

Dr D. Goldhill MA, MD, FRCA, EDIC, Consultant in Anaesthesia and Intensive Care, The Royal London Hospital, Whitechapel, London, E1 1BB, UK.

Dr S. Keegan FRCA, Specialist Registrar in Anaesthesia, Northern General Hospital, Herries Road, Sheffield, S5 7AU, UK.

Dr J. Kinsella FRCA, Senior Lecturer in Anaesthesia and Intensive Care, University Department of Anaesthesia, Glasgow Royal Infirmary, 8–16 Alexandra Parade, Glasgow, G31 2ER, UK.

Dr S.J. Mackenzie FRCA, Consultant in Intensive Care Medicine, Royal Infirmary of Edinburgh, 1 Lauriston Place, Edinburgh, EH3 9YW, UK.

Dr P. MacNaughton MD, MRCP, FRCA, Consultant in Anaesthesia and Intensive Care, Derriford Hospital, Derriford, Plymouth, PL6 8DH, UK.

Dr G.F. Mandersloot FRCA, Consultant in Anaesthesia and Intensive Care, The Royal London Hospital, Whitechapel, London, E1 1BB, UK.

Dr R. Meacher MRCP, FRCA, Consultant in Intensive Care Medicine, Charing Cross Hospital, Fulham Palace Road, London, W6 8RF, UK.

Dr G. Morgan FRCA, FRCP, Consultant in Anaesthesia and Intensive Care, Royal Cornwall Hospitals Trust, Truro, Cornwall, TR1 3LJ, UK.

Dr J. Nolan FRCA, Consultant in Anaesthesia and Intensive Care Medicine, Royal United Hospital, Combe Park, Bath, BA1 3NG, UK.

Dr J. Paddle FRCA, Specialist Registrar in Intensive Care Medicine, Royal Cornwall Hospital, Truro, Cornwall, TR1 3LJ, UK.

Dr P. Phipps FRACP, PhD, Consultant in Intensive Care and Respiratory Medicine, Royal Prince Alfred Hospital, Missenden Road, Sydney, New South Wales, 2050, Australia.

Ms T. Quasim FRCS, Senior House Officer in Anaesthesia, University Department of Anaesthesia, Glasgow Royal Infirmary, 8–16 Alexandra Parade, Glasgow, G31 2ER, UK.

Dr S. Ridley MD, FRCA, Consultant in Anaesthesia and Intensive Care, Norfolk and Norwich University NHS Trust, Colney Lane, Norwich, NR4 7UY, UK.

Dr A.G. Saayman FRCA, Special Registrar in Anaesthesia and Intensive Care, University Hospital of Wales, Heath Park, Cardiff, South Glamorgan, CF14 4XW, UK.

Dr C. Scott FRCA, Consultant in Anaesthesia and Intensive Care, Northern General Hospital, Herries Road, Sheffield, S5 7AU, UK.

Dr D. Sim MRCP, FRCA, Specialist Registrar in Anaesthesia, Royal Cornwall Hospital, Truro, Cornwall, TR1 3LJ, UK.

Dr G.B. Smith BM, FRCA, FRCP, Consultant in Intensive Care Medicine and Honorary Senior Lecturer in Critical Care, Department of Intensive Care Medicine, Portsmouth Hospitals NHS Trust, Queen Alexandra Hospital, Portsmouth, PO6 3LY, UK.

Dr B.L. Taylor BSc, FRCA, FJFICM, Consultant in Intensive Care Medicine, Department of Intensive Care Medicine, Portsmouth Hospitals NHS Trust, Queen Alexandra Hospital, Portsmouth, PO6 3LY, UK.

Dr C. Waldmann MA, FRCA, EDIC, Consultant in Anaesthesia and Intensive Care Medicine, Intensive Care Unit, Royal Berkshire Hospital, London Road, Reading, Berks, RG1 5AN, UK.

Dr D. Watson BSc (Hons), FRCA, Consultant and Senior Lecturer in Intensive Care Medicine, Anaesthetic Laboratory, St Bartholomew's Hospital, Little Britain, West Smithfield, London, EC1A 7BE, UK.

Dr J. Wigfull MRCP, FRCA, Lecturer in Anaesthesia, Academic Unit of Anaesthesia, Leeds General Infirmary, Great George Street, Leeds, LS1 3EX, UK.

Dr W. Woodward FRCA, Consultant in Anaesthesia and Intensive Care, Royal Cornwall Hospital, Truro, Cornwall, TR1 3LJ, UK.

Dr G. Wray FRCA, Consultant and Honorary Senior Lecturer in Anaesthesia and Intensive Care Medicine, Anaesthetic Laboratory, St Bartholomew's Hospital, Little Britain, West Smithfield, London, EC1A 7BE, UK.

HAEMODYNAMIC DYSFUNCTION AFTER ABDOMINAL AORTIC ANEURYSM REPAIR

M Blunt & N Barber

CASE SCENARIO

A 72-year-old man is admitted directly to the intensive care unit (ICU) following emergency abdominal aortic aneurysm repair. On his arrival in ICU, his systolic blood pressure is 115 mmHg but falls to 85 mmHg over the next 15 min. Intra-operatively he lost an estimated 4000 ml blood during a 4-h operation. His wife informs you that he had a 'heart attack' 3 years ago and can now only walk half a mile before getting chest pain. He takes aspirin and atenolol, and uses a glyceryl trinitrate spray about three times a week. He has no other significant medical history. He had been conscious on arrival at the Accident and Emergency Department but had a tachycardia (120 beats.min^{-1}) and hypotension (systolic arterial pressure 90 mmHg).

DEFINITION AND DESCRIPTION OF THE PROBLEM

Hypotension is defined as a systolic arterial blood pressure of less than 90 mmHg in a previously normotensive patient, or a fall in systolic arterial blood pressure of more than 25% of the patient's usual blood pressure. Hypotension is clinically significant if vital organ perfusion is compromised (e.g. myocardial ischaemia, oliguria and confusion). Patients presenting with a ruptured abdominal aortic aneurysm often have a number of pre-existing problems that add to the high operative mortality associated with haemorrhagic shock and lower torso ischaemia. These include increasing age, cardiovascular and cerebrovascular disease, smoking-related respiratory disease, diabetes mellitus and renal disease. In order to minimise organ dysfunction secondary to hypoperfusion, blood pressure should be maintained at or close to the patient's normal value. The usual systolic blood pressure may be obtained from old hospital notes or the general practitioner records, but if these sources are unavailable an educated guess is required. Normal systolic blood pressure in patients over 50 years of age varies between 120 and 150 mmHg. However, in patients with ischaemic heart disease and peripheral vascular disease, a relatively non-compliant vascular system will be associated with a higher blood pressure and a target pressure of 150 mmHg should be set.

PATHOPHYSIOLOGY OF THE PROBLEM

Since

$$\text{mean arterial pressure} = \text{cardiac output} \times \text{systemic vascular resistance}$$

and

$$\text{cardiac output} = \text{stroke volume} \times \text{heart rate,}$$

hypotension may result from reduced heart rate, stroke volume or systemic vascular resistance. However, it is sometimes difficult to establish which parameter is the most deranged. The heart rate may be easily obtained from the continuously monitored electrocardiogram (ECG). In a patient with a history of ischaemic heart disease, a rate of 60–80 beats.min^{-1} permits the maintenance of cardiac output while minimising myocardial work. Drugs affecting the cardiovascular system, such as atenolol, may blunt physiological responses and impair the ability to compensate for hypovolaemia.

A low stroke volume may be caused by changes in preload, myocardial contractility or afterload. Starling described the relationship between preload (initial myofibril length) and the force of contraction. The length of the cardiac muscle fibres at the start of contraction is related to the end-diastolic ventricular volume, which is mainly dependent on venous return. Venous return is reduced by hypovolaemia, head-up posture, increased intra-thoracic pressure (e.g. tension pneumothorax, positive pressure ventilation), venodilating drugs (e.g. nitrates) or cardiac tamponade. Central venous pressure (CVP) can be used as an index of right ventricular preload and, with normal cardiac function, will also reflect left ventricular preload. However, right atrial pressures do not reflect left heart function in patients with left ventricular failure, severe bundle branch block, pulmonary hypertension, chronic pulmonary disease, interstitial pulmonary oedema and valvular heart disease; here the pulmonary capillary wedge pressure (PCWP) may be used as an estimate of left ventricular preload.

Myocardial contractility is reduced by hypoxaemia, hypothermia, hypercapnia, ischaemic heart disease, myocardial infarction, acidosis, electrolyte imbalances and negatively inotropic drugs (e.g. inhalational anaesthetic agents and anti-arrhythmic drugs). Afterload is the ventricular wall tension required to eject the stroke volume during systole; increased afterload results in increased myocardial work and oxygen consumption and a decreased stroke volume. Afterload is increased by increased ventricular volume (according to Laplace's law), decreased elasticity of the large blood vessels (e.g. with age), aortic stenosis and increased systemic vascular resistance. Systemic vascular resistance is determined by the diameter of arterioles and is under both neural and humoral control.

Hypovolaemia or myocardial dysfunction is the most likely cause for the hypotension seen in this patient. He has sustained large, peri-operative blood loss (4000 ml recorded losses in theatre) and is likely to have both consumptive and dilutional coagulopathies; these will be exacerbated by hypothermia. He has a history of ischaemic heart disease and may have developed myocardial dysfunction secondary to the increased afterload produced by the cross clamp applied to his aorta during surgery. During surgery, reperfusion of the lower limbs results in the release of lactic acid which depresses myocardial function. Similarly, hypothermia due to prolonged peri-operative exposure and large volume intravenous infusions will also depress the myocardium. Circulatory compensation mechanisms, particularly tachycardia and elevated systemic resistance, increase myocardial work and oxygen requirements at the very time that supply is threatened; this can also worsen myocardial dysfunction. Although not present in this patient, epidural anaesthesia can contribute to hypotension by sympathetic blockade.

THERAPEUTIC GOALS

The therapeutic goals in this patient include:

1. The prompt reversal of hypotension to avoid hypoperfusion of vital organs.

2. The empirical treatment of hypotension, while instituting further monitoring to identify precisely the most prominent cause.

3. The frequent assessment of the patient's response to treatment.

THERAPEUTIC OPTIONS BASED ON PHYSIOLOGICAL AND PHARMACOLOGICAL EFFECTS

The initial approach to the patient should follow the airway breathing circulation (ABC) algorithm developed for adult cardiac life support.

Airway

Although the patient has been transferred from the operating room, intubated, ventilated and sedated, the position of the tracheal tube should be checked by auscultation of the chest and chest X-ray.

Breathing

Breathing is maintained by controlled ventilation, adjusting the F_iO_2 to maintain the P_aO_2 between 9 and 12 kPa. If a tension pneumothorax is suspected of causing the hypotension, treatment involves immediate decompression by a large bore cannula in the anterior, second intercostal space at the mid-clavicular line, followed by formal tube thoracocentesis.

Circulation

The circulation can be assessed clinically by the rate, rhythm and volume of the pulse. A difference >5°C between the peripheral temperature (hand skin probe) with the core temperature (oesophageal or nasal probe) suggests significant peripheral vasoconstriction. Pale, cool peripheries, and oliguria (urine output < $0.5\,ml.kg^{-1}.h^{-1}$) indicate hypoperfusion. The arterial line inserted in theatre allows direct, continuous measurement of blood pressure, but should be checked for accuracy by re-zeroing and examining the waveform for damping, as both could cause inaccuracies in measurement.

In establishing the cause of hypotension, the assessment of ventricular preload by CVP or pulmonary artery catheter (PAC) is crucial. CVP is increased by raised intra-thoracic pressure, impaired cardiac function, venoconstriction and circulatory overload. The effect of a 250-ml fluid challenge on the CVP reading is more useful than its absolute value. A smaller bolus (100 ml) should be used if it is likely that the hypotension is of cardiac origin. A volume challenge causing a persistent rise in CVP of over 3 mmHg suggests a well-filled circulating volume or poor ventricular function in a normovolaemic patient. Hypovolaemia is suggested if the fluid challenge increases the CVP value by <3 mmHg or causes a rise sustained for less than 10–15 min. If CVP measurement does not help in assessing ventricular preload, the use of a PAC or transoesophageal Doppler probe may provide further guidance.

Pulmonary artery catheter

In some clinical situations, CVP values do not correlate with left atrial pressures (see above). In the described patient, this is a consideration because his previous myocardial infarction may have altered left ventricular compliance. PCWP is measured by wedging a flow-directed balloon-tipped catheter into a small pulmonary artery. When wedged, a continuous column of blood connects the catheter tip to the left atrium via the pulmonary capillaries and veins, and the measured pressure reflects left ventricular preload in most situations. Values should be interpreted with caution in left ventricular failure, mitral valve disease, raised intra-thoracic pressure, non–compliant left ventricles and aortic regurgitation. As with the CVP, response to a fluid challenge is more helpful than absolute values, but initial PCWP target values of 15–18 mmHg are appropriate. PACs allow intermittent or continuous measurement of cardiac output by thermodilution. However, their use in critically ill patients is controversial. Complications of their use include arrhythmias, catheter knotting, pulmonary infarction, pulmonary artery rupture and infection.

Transoesophageal Doppler

Transoesophageal Doppler ultrasound is an increasingly popular alternative to PAC insertion and is a less-invasive way of assessing circulatory volume status and cardiac function. Blood flow in the descending thoracic aorta is monitored via a probe placed in the distal oesophagus and gives a characteristic waveform (Figure 1.1).

The area under each waveform (i.e. the stroke distance) represents the stroke volume with 85% accuracy when corrected for patient's age, weight and height. The peak velocity measures myocardial contractility and normally declines with age. The flow time corrected for heart rate (FTc) is inversely proportional to systemic vascular resistance and is therefore low in hypovolaemia and arterial constriction, and gives a guide to fluid status. A fluid challenge increases FTc and stroke distance in hypovolaemia, but reduces peak velocity in poor ventricular function. Measurement

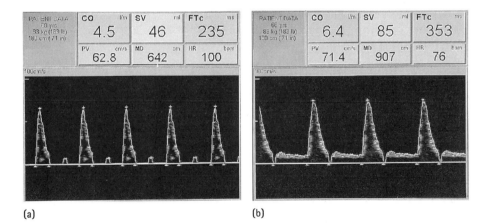

(a)   (b)

Figure 1.1 – Transoesophageal Doppler monitor screen demonstrating a patient: (a) with hypotension due to hypovolaemia. In this patient, the SV is relatively low (46 ml) and is associated with low FTc (235 ms) and the waveform can be seen to be peaked and narrow suggesting that flow is only occurring in the earliest part of systole. HR is also elevated; however, the PV is maintained at the near-normal for this patient suggesting poor contractility is not a problem. (b) following fluid resuscitation. After appropriate volume loading, the CO and SV have improved substantially with a reflex fall in HR. FTc is now at the normally targeted value (350–400 ms) and the waveform looks wider and fuller. PV has increased slightly showing that the heart was capable of better contractility with increased preload.

Abbreviations: CO, cardiac output; SV, stroke volume; FTc, flow time corrected; PV, peak velocity; MD, mean distance; HR, heart rate.

of stroke volume before and after the administration of a fluid challenge is a safe and effective method to evaluate post–operative hypotension. Fluid boluses should be continued until the rise in stroke volume is less than 10%, implying that the slope of the preload–contractility curve has flattened. Although extremely safe in normal usage, transoesophageal Doppler is contraindicated in patients with oesophageal pathology or marked coagulopathy. There are few reported complications even with prolonged use.

Hypovolaemia

Patients may be hypovolaemic following surgery due to continuing or inadequate replacement of losses, or redistribution of intravascular volume. To enable rapid fluid resuscitation, at least two large venous cannulae should be sited. In patients with difficult venous access, insertion of a PAC introducer into a major vein provides wide bore venous access and allows subsequent flotation of a PAC if required. The primary objective is to restore the circulating volume as guided by the patient's response to fluid boluses (i.e. changes in pulse rate, blood pressure, peripheral perfusion, urine output, CVP and PCWP). A combination of colloids (i.e. gelatins, starches or albumin) and isotonic crystalloids can be used. Debate continues as to the 'best' fluid for resuscitation and maintenance in critically ill patients and, in the absence of strong evidence, no firm recommendations can be made. However, it must be remembered that colloids will expand the intravascular volume three times more than an equivalent volume of crystalloid due to their tendency to remain in the intravascular space. The results of blood tests taken on ICU admission (e.g. full blood count, haematocrit and coagulation) will determine blood products requirement. Transfusion is rarely indicated when the haemoglobin concentration is over $10\,\mathrm{g.dl}^{-1}$. However, in this patient, an inability to correct hypovolaemia may suggest ongoing bleeding, in which case transfusion should be instigated. Transfusion is almost always indicated when the haemoglobin concentration is below $6\,\mathrm{g.dl}^{-1}$. The platelet count should be kept above $50 \times 10^9\,\mathrm{l}^{-1}$ as platelet function may be impaired by aspirin therapy in this patient. Activated partial thromboplastin time (APTT) and prothrombin time (PT) greater than 1.5 times the normal values require correction with fresh frozen plasma (FFP). Continued coagulopathy may require cryoprecipitate, especially if fibrinogen levels are less than $0.8\,\mathrm{g.l}^{-1}$. Antifibrinolytic agents (e.g. aprotinin) may occasionally have a role. Fluid warming and warm air blankets will correct hypothermia. As the patient warms, there is an initial rise in lactate representing washout from previously underperfused tissues and an increased need for further intravascular volume expansion as the peripheries dilate. Sympathomimetics with vasoconstricting action are occasionally required to increase vascular tone transiently while fluid resuscitation occurs. However, long term or high doses of vasoconstrictors must be avoided in hypovolaemic patients. An urgent surgical review should be sought if abdominal girth increases or there is continuing blood loss into surgical drains, as a second laparotomy may be required.

Myocardial dysfunction

If the hypotension persists despite adequate circulating volume (as indicated by CVP and PCWP) and there is no suspicion of sepsis, the cause is likely to be cardiogenic. Arrhythmias, myocardial infarction (old or new) and ongoing ischaemia (ST segment depression, T-wave inversion) can be assessed by a 12-lead ECG performed on admission to ICU. Biochemical abnormalities (e.g. hypokalaemia and hypomagnesaemia) predispose to arrhythmias and require correction as arrhythmias reduce ventricular filling and, hence, cardiac output. If arrhythmias persist despite high normal serum potassium (4.5–5.5 mmol.l^{-1}) and magnesium (1.0 mmol.l^{-1}) levels, mechanical stimulation should be excluded by withdrawing the CVP catheter and PAC into the superior vena cava. If this fails to correct the rhythm, direct current (DC) cardioversion (for atrial fibrillation, ventricular tachycardia), pacing (for complete heart block) or an amiodarone infusion may be indicated.

Laboratory measurement of cardiac enzymes may help to confirm or refute suspected myocardial infarction. Myocardial specific creatinine kinase (CKMB) rises 6 h after myocardial infarction. Troponin I is a more sensitive and specific marker of acute myocardial infarction than CKMB; it is normally undetectable and rises 6 h after myocardial infarction. It peaks at 12 h and falls between 5 and 9 days after the

Table 1.1 – Cardiovascular drugs commonly used in patients following emergency abdominal aneurysm surgery.

Drug	Dose (μg.kg^{-1}.min^{-1})	Action	Site of action
Epinephrine	0.01–1.0	+++ heart rate +++ contractility ++ arterial constriction	Primarily β1- and β2- with some α-agonism at high dose
Norepinephrine	0.01–1.0	+/− heart rate + contractility +++ arterial constriction	Almost exclusively α-agonism
Dopamine	1–20	++ heart rate ++ contractility ++ arterial vasoconstriction	β-agonism at lower doses with increasing α-action at higher doses. Renal effect is seen experimentally but has little proven benefit in patients
Dopexamine	0.5	++ heart rate + contractility ++ splanchnic and renal dilatation	β2-agonism and DA-1 agonism with some evidence of benefit on urine output
Enoximone	0.5–1.0* then 5–20	+ heart rate +++ contractility +++ arterial dilatation	Phosphodiesterase inhibition increasing cAMP levels
Glyceryl trinitrate	0.2–5.0	+++ venodilatation + arterial dilatation	Veno- and vasodilatation by nitric oxide production

*μg.kg^{-1} bolus.

infarct. Fibrinolytic therapy is contraindicated after surgery and the treatment of myocardial infarction or ischaemia is, therefore, supportive.

The initial management of cardiac dysfunction involves optimisation of preload by fluid challenges to achieve a CVP or PCWP of 16–18 mmHg. This is followed by vasoactive drug support using noradrenaline, adrenaline or dobutamine, to achieve a mean blood pressure of 70–80 mmHg. Haemodynamic monitoring (PAC or transoesophageal Doppler) helps guide choice of inotrope (Table 1.1).

Sympathomimetics increase vascular tone by action on peripheral α-receptors, and heart rate and contractility by their effects on cardiac α- and β-receptors. Phosphodiesterase inhibitors (e.g. milrinone, amrinone and enoximone) improve contractility by increasing cyclic adenosine monophosphate levels but also cause vasodilatation. Vasodilators help decrease PCWP in the presence of pulmonary oedema and improve cardiac output by reducing afterload.

USUAL OUTCOME

Emergency aortic aneurysm repair is associated with 50–60% mortality; pre-operative hypotension, intraperitoneal rupture, pre-operative coagulopathy and pre-operative cardiac arrest have been identified as independent predictors of increased mortality.

KEY LEARNING POINTS

1. The intravascular volume should be normalised by the infusion of intravenous fluids.

2. The response of CVP and PCWP to a fluid bolus is a useful indicator of volume and cardiac status.

3. Early surgical review is required if hypovolaemia and hypotension persists despite apparently adequate fluid replacement.

4. Myocardial contractility and vascular tone may require support with inotropic or vasoconstrictor drugs.

Further reading

1. Sielenkamper A, Sibbald WJ. Pathophysiology of hypotension. In Webb AR, Shapiro MJ, Singer M, Suter PM (eds), *Oxford Textbook of Critical Care*. Oxford: Oxford Medical Publications, 1999: 215–28.

2. Stainsby D, MacLennan S, Hamilton PJ. Management of massive blood loss: a template guideline. *British Journal of Anaesthesia* 2000; **85**: 487–91.

3. Turton EP, Scott DJ, Delbridge M, Snowden S, Kester RC. Ruptured abdominal aortic aneurysm: a novel method of outcome prediction using neural network technology. *European Journal of Vascular and Endovascular Surgery* 2000; **19**: 184–9.

4. Milner QJ, Burchett KR. Long term survival following emergency abdominal aortic aneurysm repair. *Anaesthesia* 2000; **55**: 432–5.

2

TRAUMATIC LUNG CONTUSION

J Paddle & P MacNaughton

CASE SCENARIO

A 23-year-old male is admitted after a motor vehicle crash in which he sustained chest and abdominal injuries including multiple left-sided rib fractures and a ruptured spleen. He required an emergency splenectomy, and was transfused 10 units of blood prior to his admission to the intensive care unit (ICU), where he remains intubated and ventilated. Five hours after admission to ICU, his blood pressure and pulse are stable, but his arterial oxygen saturation has fallen from 96% to 85% despite 100% inspired oxygen.

DEFINITION AND DESCRIPTION OF THE PROBLEM

This patient has life threatening hypoxaemic respiratory failure, which needs to be corrected urgently. A number of mechanisms may cause respiratory failure in ventilated patients, who have suffered severe chest trauma; these include:

1. *Early complications of chest trauma:*

    - airway injury (e.g. trachea, bronchus and alveolus);

    - pneumothorax and haemothorax;

    - flail chest (i.e. three or more consecutive ribs with each broken in at least two places);

    - pulmonary contusion;

    - diaphragmatic rupture.

2. *Delayed complications of chest trauma:*

    - late presentation of acute complications listed above;

    - atelectasis;

- nosocomial pneumonia;

- acute respiratory distress syndrome (ARDS);

- pulmonary oedema due to cardiac contusion.

3. *Other causes of hypoxaemia in ventilated patients:*

- problems with tracheal tubes (e.g. misplacement, kinking and obstruction by secretions/blood);

- incorrect ventilator settings;

- inadequate sedation and analgesia resulting in patient–ventilator dysynchrony;

- mechanical faults with the ventilator;

- alterations in positive end-expiratory pressure (PEEP) or F_iO_2.

PATHOLOGY AND PATHOPHYSIOLOGY OF RESPIRATORY FAILURE FOLLOWING CHEST TRAUMA

Respiratory failure can be classified as hypoxaemic ($P_aO_2 < 8\,kPa$ or $60\,mmHg$), hypercapnic ($P_aCO_2 > 6.7\,kPa$ or $50\,mmHg$) or mixed. Hypoxaemia usually arises from ventilation : perfusion ($V:Q$) mismatch, the most severe form being intra-pulmonary shunt in which areas of the lung are perfused, but not ventilated. Following chest trauma, shunt may be caused by airway obstruction due to secretions or blood, atelectasis and alveolar haemorrhage caused by lung contusion or alveolar flooding due to pulmonary oedema (as in ARDS or severe cardiac contusion). Hypercapnia results from inadequate alveolar minute ventilation, which may be due to inadequate respiratory drive (e.g. associated head trauma or excessive opiate analgesia), disruption of chest wall mechanics (e.g. painful rib fractures, flail chest or haemo/pneumothorax) or respiratory muscle fatigue due to excessive work of breathing.

The time of onset of respiratory failure following chest trauma will vary. Early hypoxaemia is usually due to pneumothorax and/or haemothorax, requiring urgent treatment as part of the initial resuscitation. Hypoxaemia, following lung contusion and rib fractures, may initially be mild but may subsequently worsen. Inadequate analgesia for rib fractures will restrict breathing and impair cough, leading to atelectasis, retention of secretions and nosocomial pneumonia.

Multiple rib fractures can result in a flail segment, which can be lateral, with fractures affecting at least three consecutive ribs in two different places, or central, where the sternum forms part of the flail segment. During spontaneous respiration, the loss of chest wall integrity results in paradoxical movement of the flail segment, with inward movement on inspiration. Hypoxaemia arises in part from atelectasis, but is mainly due to the underlying lung contusion, which may be severe. If the patient cannot increase minute ventilation in other uninjured areas of the lung, hypercapnia will occur. This may be delayed due to the development of respiratory muscle fatigue. The application of positive pressure (e.g. PEEP or continuous positive airway pressure (CPAP)) prevents paradoxical movement and improves respiratory function.

Major chest trauma invariably results in an acute lung injury (ALI) characterised by impaired gas exchange associated with bilateral airspace shadowing on chest X-ray. In many patients, this is severe and fulfils the criteria for ARDS (Table 2.1).

Table 2.1 – Diagnostic criteria for ALI and ARDS.

Acute onset.
Bilateral infiltrates on chest X-ray.
Pulmonary artery wedge pressure $\leqslant 18$ mmHg, or the absence of clinical evidence of left atrial hypertension.
ALI present, if $P_aO_2 : F_iO_2$ ratio is <300 mmHg (40.0 kPa)
ARDS present, if $P_aO_2 : F_iO_2$ ratio is $\leqslant 200$ mmHg (26.7 kPa).

Although ARDS may arise from many different precipitating conditions, it is characterised by refractory hypoxaemia due to pulmonary oedema caused by increased pulmonary capillary permeability.

At the site of pulmonary contusion, there is an early and localised parenchymal injury that produces interstitial oedema and haemorrhage. This results in a diffuse pulmonary and systemic inflammatory response, which is mediated by activation of circulating neutrophils and alveolar macrophages, and results in the production of cytokines and other pro-inflammatory substances. Other pulmonary and non-pulmonary factors may stimulate this response including pulmonary aspiration, infection, circulatory shock, massive blood transfusion and fat embolus. The interaction of activated neutrophils with the vascular endothelium in the lungs results in damage to the alveolar–capillary barrier, leading to pulmonary interstitial and alveolar oedema. Alveolar flooding and atelectasis of dependent lung areas underlying oedematous, dense lung causes a marked increase in intra-pulmonary shunt associated with a reduction in lung compliance. Pulmonary hypertension may arise from pulmonary vasoconstriction and micro-vascular occlusion. ARDS represents the pulmonary manifestation of a systemic inflammatory disorder and associated multi-organ dysfunction is common.

Although the chest X-ray typically shows diffuse airspace shadowing, CT-scan studies reveal that the injured lung can be divided into three broad regions:

1. apparently normally ventilated lung,

2. atelectatic regions which can be potentially opened ('recruited'),

3. consolidated non-recruitable lung (Figure 2.1a and b).

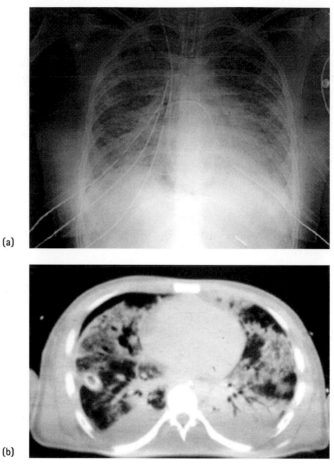

(a)

(b)

Figure 2.1 – Radiographic changes of ARDS following chest trauma. (a) The X-ray shows diffuse airspace shadowing. Bilateral chest drains are visible. (b) The CT scan reveals distinct areas of apparently normal lung and consolidated lung tissue. Note that the anterior right-sided pneumothorax is not visible on the chest X-ray. A right-sided chest drain and bilateral small posterior effusions are visible.

Ventilatory strategies in ARDS aim to open the recruitable lung, thereby improving gas exchange without over-distending the normal lung. There is considerable experimental and clinical evidence that inappropriate setting of ventilators can induce a lung injury indistinguishable from other causes of ARDS. This is termed ventilation-induced lung injury and lung damage appears to be caused both from excessive tidal volume (volutrauma) and from the inflammatory response that is induced, if cyclical opening and closure of atelectatic lung occurs during tidal ventilation. Prolonged exposure to high-inspired oxygen concentrations may also promote damage by increasing oxygen-derived free-radical injury.

THERAPEUTIC GOALS

The therapeutic goals in this patient include:

1. The priority is to recognise and treat hypoxaemia according to basic principles (i.e. airway, breathing and circulation). In most patients, the target is to maintain $P_aO_2 > 8\,kPa$ and $S_aO_2 > 92\%$.

2. The most appropriate mode of ventilatory support should be chosen, which improves gas exchange and minimises complications.

3. Effective analgesia should be provided, in order to reduce the risk of exacerbating respiratory failure.

4. Ensure that complications following multiple trauma (e.g. fat embolism after long bone fractures and neurogenic pulmonary oedema after severe head injury) are prevented or promptly recognised and managed effectively.

THERAPEUTIC OPTIONS BASED ON PHYSIOLOGICAL AND PHARMACOLOGICAL EFFECTS

Treatment of immediate causes of hypoxia

Assessment includes taking a relevant history and thorough physical examination, concentrating on correct management of the airway, breathing and circulation. The tracheal tube may become misplaced, kinked or blocked by foreign bodies including blood and mucus. Endobronchial intubation is common following emergency intubation, and the correct position of the tube should be confirmed by inspection, auscultation of the breath sounds and review of the chest X-ray. To confirm that the tracheal tube lumen is patent, a suction catheter should be passed. If doubt remains, the tracheal tube should be replaced. Fibreoptic bronchoscopy may be indicated for bronchial toilet and to assess possible airway injury (see below).

Pneumothorax is usually recognised and treated during the initial assessment of the patient, but presentation may be delayed. Instituting positive-pressure ventilation may convert a simple pneumothorax to a tension pneumothorax. Previously inserted thoracic drains may become displaced or blocked. In ventilated patients, a pneumothorax may be difficult to recognise, as the clinical signs may not be obvious. The typical chest X-ray signs of a pneumothorax may be absent (e.g. there may be no clear lung edge visible). However, a pneumothorax should be suspected if the chest X-ray shows a clearly demarcated area of increased lung translucency or the deep sulcus sign (i.e. a depressed, flattened diaphragm with associated thoracic hyperlucency). A tension pneumothorax will cause haemodynamic compromise with normal or high central venous pressures, impaired gas exchange and increased ventilator airway pressures. In the stable patient, a CT scan may confirm the diagnosis of a simple pneumothorax, but needle thoracocentesis, with subsequent tube thoracocentesis, should be performed immediately in patients with signs of a tension pneumothorax.

A persistent air leak from a correctly positioned chest drain suggests a bronchopleural fistula. The leak can be quantified by comparing the inspired and expired minute volumes recorded by the ventilator. Most bronchopleural fistulae heal with conservative management, usually when positive-pressure ventilation is discontinued. During ventilatory support, mean airway pressures should be kept to a minimum to reduce the leak. Major airway injuries are rare, but should be considered when there is a persistent pneumothorax with a large air leak and associated mediastinal and subcutaneous emphysema. These require surgical repair.

A haemothorax is common in the presence of rib fractures and may be associated with a pneumothorax. Treatment is by drainage using a large bore chest drain. If bleeding continues, thoracotomy may be required.

Patients with flail segments are at high risk of developing respiratory failure. Effective analgesia may prevent deterioration in respiratory function, although some form of positive-pressure ventilation, either by face mask or tracheal intubation, will usually be required to reduce the paradoxical chest wall motion and improve respiratory function.

Choice of ventilatory support

The method of respiratory support for patients with acute hypoxaemic respiratory failure depends primarily on the severity of the respiratory failure. Methods range from simple oxygen therapy to advanced ventilation techniques (Table 2.2).

Conventional ventilation

Modern ICU ventilators can be classified into those that deliver a preset tidal volume (e.g. volume control and synchronised intermittent mandatory ventilation (SIMV)) or those that deliver a preset inspiratory pressure (e.g. pressure control

Table 2.2 – Options for respiratory support in hypoxaemic respiratory failure.

Method	Example
Face mask oxygen	Nasal cannulae, face mask, reservoir face mask, CPAP
Non-invasive ventilation	Pressure control or support
Volume-controlled ventilation	Volume control, SIMV*
Pressure-controlled ventilation	Pressure control, pressure control-IRV**
Posture	Prone ventilation
Inhalation therapy	NO, prostacyclin
Extra-corporeal techniques	Extra-corporeal membrane oxygenation
Advanced techniques under investigation	High frequency oscillator ventilation, liquid ventilation

*Synchronised intermittent mandatory ventilation.
**Inverse ratio ventilation.

and pressure support). In modes with a preset inspiratory pressure, the delivered tidal volume will vary with the respiratory system mechanical characteristics (i.e. resistance and compliance) and the patient's respiratory efforts. A mode that delivers a preset tidal volume between 8 and $10\,\mathrm{ml.kg}^{-1}$ is commonly used as the initial mode for adults with acute respiratory failure. This results in predictable minute ventilation, CO_2 clearance and pH control. In patients with ARDS, poor lung compliance will result in high airway pressures, which may exacerbate the lung injury. Pressure control has become popular in the management of ARDS, as it minimises peak airway pressures. Current guidelines are to limit airway pressures to less than 30–35 cmH_2O in order to reduce ventilator-induced lung injury. However, appropriate use of pressure control requires vigilance to avoid excessive tidal volumes. The ARDS network has demonstrated that low-tidal-volume ventilation ($<6\,\mathrm{ml.kg}^{-1}$) is associated with an improved outcome when compared to high volume ventilation. Respiratory acidosis can be minimised by increasing respiratory rate (up to 30 breaths.min^{-1}) and by sodium bicarbonate infusion. The ARDS network protocol, which uses volume control, has been adopted by a number of centres as the current optimal method for ventilatory support in ARDS.

High-inspired oxygen tensions may be ineffective in improving hypoxaemia in ARDS. Oxygenation will be improved, quite often dramatically, if atelectatic areas of the lung can be recruited. The application of PEEP is the most common method for recruiting collapsed lung. Most patients start on 5 cmH_2O of PEEP, which is then adjusted according to the change in P_aO_2. Typically levels of up to 10 cmH_2O are used, although up to 20 cmH_2O may be required. The full recruitment effect of PEEP may not be apparent for several hours. The application of PEEP will increase airway pressures, which may result in lung over-distension and volutrauma. It may be necessary to reduce tidal volumes and increase frequency, following the application of PEEP, to ensure that airway pressures are kept within reasonable limits. PEEP may impair venous return, reducing cardiac output and blood pressure, particularly if the patient is hypovolaemic. A number of methods have been used to optimise PEEP. Adjusting the level of PEEP, so that measured lung compliance is highest, implies that ventilation is occurring on the optimal part of the lung pressure–volume curve. If cardiac output is monitored, PEEP can be titrated to that which results in maximum oxygen delivery. In practice, PEEP and F_iO_2 are usually adjusted empirically according to P_aO_2 while monitoring vital signs (Table 2.3).

Table 2.3 – Setting of F_iO_2 and PEEP according to ARDS Network protocol.

F_iO_2	0.3	0.4	0.5	0.6	0.7	0.8	0.9	1.0
PEEP (cmH$_2$0)	5	5–8	8–10	10	10–14	14	14–18	18–24

Target P_aO_2: 7.3–10.7 kPa (55–80 mmHg), S_aO_2: 88–95%.
Modified from Acute Respiratory Distress Syndrome Network. Ventilation with lower tidal volumes as compared to traditional volumes for acute lung injury and the acute respiratory distress syndrome. *New England Journal of Medicine* 2000; **342**: 1301–8.

Assessment of the pulmonary static pressure–volume curve may be used to guide the optimal ventilator strategy in ARDS. When the pressure–volume curve is analysed, a low–inflection point, marking an increase in compliance, may be identified. This is thought to represent the airway pressure at which recruitment of closed areas of lung is starting to occur. A high–inflection point may also be identified, when lung compliance abruptly decreases representing lung over-distension. It has been suggested that optimal ventilator setting is with a PEEP level set above the pressure of the lower-inflection point and the maximum end-inspiratory pause pressure set just below the upper-inflection point. This typically results in PEEP levels of around $18\,cmH_2O$ with an inspiratory pressure of approximately $30\,cmH_2O$. However, measuring the static pressure–volume curve requires equipment that is not readily available in the majority of ICUs with the result that the measurement is not widely performed.

Prolonging the inspiratory phase of ventilation, by the application of an end-inspiratory pause, may be used to improve oxygenation. This is achieved by changing the ratio of inspiratory to expiratory time ($I:E$ ratio) from the normal $1:2$. Inverse ratio ventilation (IRV) describes the situation in which inspiration lasts longer than expiration. Increasing inspiratory time elevates mean airway pressure, which may recruit alveoli and keep them open. Parts of the lung with long-time constants are also more effectively ventilated reducing $V:Q$ mismatch. However, reducing expiratory time may not allow complete expiration. This results in dynamic hyper-inflation and the risk of barotrauma and haemodynamic compromise. If dynamic hyperinflation occurs, alveolar pressure at end expiration is increased above the level of PEEP set on the ventilator. This additional pressure is termed intrinsic or auto-PEEP, which should be monitored when IRV is applied. IRV is more safely applied with pressure-controlled ventilation than volume-controlled ventilation as the set inspiratory pressure will limit dynamic hyperinflation.

Other ventilation strategies

Changing the position of the patient from supine to prone may result in a dramatic improvement in oxygenation in ARDS. The prone position improves ventilation of the dorsal, atelectatic areas of the lung, reducing $V:Q$ mismatch. Patients are usually managed in the prone position for between 6 and 24 h. After returning to supine, the improvement in oxygenation is sustained in many patients, although in others there is a deterioration requiring one or more additional periods of prone therapy. Prone ventilation should be considered in all patients with ARDS, although in certain patients the practical aspects need consideration. Care is needed when turning patients to prevent accidental removal of lines and tubes, and to avoid skin pressure damage. In the trauma patient, the presence of other injuries such as spinal cord injuries or external fixator devices may preclude its use.

CT-scan studies have revealed that some areas of atelectatic lung do not open until airway pressures between 40 and $60\,cmH_2O$ are applied. Such pressures cannot be applied for prolonged periods during mechanical ventilation without adverse effects. However, the use of high pressures for short periods has been proposed as an effective lung recruitment manoeuvre. In some patients, these techniques may result in a sustained improvement in oxygenation, although they should be used with caution and may be contraindicated in patients with chest trauma due to the risk of producing a pneumothorax in already damaged lung.

Applying ventilatory support in patients with a large bronchopleural fistula can be challenging, as the applied minute ventilation will leak preferentially through the fistula resulting in inadequate ventilation of the contralateral lung. One approach is to isolate the two lungs with a double lumen endobronchial tube and to ventilate the lungs independently using two ventilators. The diffusely injured lung receives conventional ventilation, and the lung with the fistula is ventilated with low-airway pressures to minimise the leak.

Extra-corporeal membrane oxygenation describes the use of a heart–lung bypass machine to augment gas exchange in patients with severe acute respiratory failure. Two randomised controlled trials in adults with ARDS have failed to show any benefit from this highly invasive technique, and there is little place for this therapy in light of the improved outcome with current methods of conventional respiratory support.

High frequency oscillator ventilation is a mode of ventilatory support that achieves gas exchange with high frequency low-amplitude pressure oscillations. It uses respiratory rates between 60 and 900 breaths.min^{-1} and produces high mean airway pressures with low-tidal volumes between 1 and 2 ml.kg^{-1}. As the tidal volumes are less than dead space, limited gas exchange can occur by bulk flow and a number of other mechanisms have been proposed. Most experience with this technique is in neonatal and paediatric respiratory failure, where it appears to be very successful. Some preliminary studies in adult ARDS have suggested that high frequency oscillation may be successful in improving gas exchange when conventional support has failed. As this technique combines a high mean airway pressure with minimal tidal volume, it is postulated that it will maximise lung recruitment while minimising ventilator-induced lung injury. Results of controlled trials are awaited to establish what the role of high frequency oscillator ventilation is in the management of patients with ARDS.

Drug therapy

Nitric oxide (NO) is a potent endogenous vasodilator with a very short half-life, produced by the vascular endothelium. If used therapeutically by inhalation, it has a highly selective action on the pulmonary vasculature. Vasodilatation occurs in the blood vessels supplying the ventilated parts of the lung, thereby reducing pulmonary vascular resistance and improving $V : Q$ mismatch. Inhaled NO has been shown to temporarily improve oxygenation and reduce pulmonary arterial pressures in approximately 50% of patients with ARDS. However, the effects seem to be short lived and no reduction in mortality has been demonstrated. Inhaled NO may have a number of adverse effects including the suppression of endogenous NO production, impairment of left ventricular function, platelet dysfunction and free-radical-mediated damage. Its use cannot be recommended except for the short-term reversal of refractory hypoxaemia and the treatment of right heart failure secondary to pulmonary hypertension. Prostacyclin, when administered as a continuous aerosol, acts as a selective pulmonary vasodilator with similar effects to inhaled NO and can be used as an alternative.

Although ARDS follows a systemic inflammatory response, attempts to inhibit this process pharmacologically have proved disappointing. Anti-inflammatory therapy with agents such as corticosteroids, prostaglandin E_1 and anti-tumour necrosis factor (anti-TNF) antibody has proved ineffective. There may be a role for prolonged steroid therapy in patients who remain ventilator dependent without signs of sepsis after 7–14 days of conventional supportive treatment. In this subgroup of patients, an aggressive fibro-proliferative process may prevent recovery of lung function; such fibro-proliferation appears to be reduced by prolonged corticosteroid therapy (e.g. intravenous methylprednisolone $2\,mg.kg^{-1}.day^{-1}$ for 14 days).

Analgesia

Inadequate analgesia results in reduced tidal volumes and poor cough. Atelectasis, respiratory compromise and pneumonia may follow. In selected patients, non-steroidal anti-inflammatory drugs can be a useful adjunct, but these are rarely sufficient as the only means of pain relief. A thoracic epidural with a continuous infusion of a local anaesthetic and opioid provides excellent analgesia and often prevents deterioration of lung function. The side effects of systemic opioids, particularly sedation and respiratory depression, are largely avoided by this technique.

General measures to reduce complications

Thorough and repeated evaluation of the patient ensures that all injuries are promptly recognised and managed optimally. Vigilance is required to reduce complications such as nosocomial sepsis. The use of a short course (<72 h) of broad-spectrum antibiotics may reduce septic complications in trauma patients, but prolonged antibiotic prescription will select resistant organisms and should be avoided. Managing the patient in the semi-recumbent (e.g. 30° head-up) rather than the supine position reduces the incidence of nosocomial pneumonia. Invasive lines should be placed under strict aseptic conditions and removed promptly when they are no longer required. The early use of enteral nutrition has been shown to reduce morbidity from sepsis following major trauma and may be more successfully established if a jejunal feeding tube is placed at laparotomy.

Following splenectomy, this patient is at risk of life threatening infections from encapsulated bacteria. Life-long prophylactic antibiotic therapy will be required (e.g. amoxicillin: 250 mg daily), but immunisation against *Pneumococcus, Haemophilus* and *Meningococcus* species should be delayed until 7–10 days post-operatively to increase the likelihood of seroconversion.

USUAL OUTCOME

Immediate and early mortality is related to the severity of the initial injury. Mortality from ARDS has improved over the last decade and is between 30% and 50% for all causes, although the outcome of patients who develop ARDS following trauma is usually better. Sepsis remains the most common cause of death and measures to reduce this complication should improve outcome. Furthermore, appropriate ventilation strategies have been shown to reduce mortality.

KEY LEARNING POINTS

1. The priority is to recognise and treat hypoxaemia according to basic principles (i.e. airway, breathing and circulation). Life threatening thoracic injuries must be recognised and treated promptly.

2. Effective pain control with a thoracic epidural may prevent deterioration of respiratory function.

3. Positive-pressure ventilation will improve respiratory failure secondary to a flail segment.

4. ARDS may occur following major chest trauma; appropriate ventilation strategies include the use of low-tidal volumes and PEEP.

5. Non-invasive ventilation may be used to avoid intubation in selected patients.

Further reading

1. Sabbe MB. Recent advances in the diagnosis and treatment of thoracic injury. *Current Opinion in Critical Care* 1995; **1**: 503–8.

2. The Acute Respiratory Distress Syndrome Network. Ventilation with lower tidal volumes as compared to traditional tidal volumes for acute lung injury and the acute respiratory distress syndrome. *New England Journal of Medicine* 2000; **342**: 1301–8.

3. Tobin MJ. Advances in mechanical ventilation. *New England Journal of Medicine* 2001; **344**: 1986–96.

4. Ware LB, Matthay MA. The acute respiratory distress syndrome. *New England Journal of Medicine* 2000; **342**: 1334–49.

5. Westaby S. The pathophysiology and treatment of thoracic injuries. In Garrard C, Foëx P, Westaby S (eds), *Principles and Practice of Critical Care*. Oxford: Blackwell Science, 1997: 553–83.

6. Voggenreiter G, Neudeck F, Aufmkolk M *et al*. Intermittent prone positioning in the treatment of severe and moderate posttraumatic lung injury. *Critical Care Medicine* 1999; **27**: 2375–82.

3

RESPIRATORY FAILURE DUE TO CHRONIC OBSTRUCTIVE PULMONARY DISEASE

R T J Cree & S V Baudouin

CASE SCENARIO

A 71-year-old man with chronic obstructive pulmonary disease (COPD) is admitted to the Accident and Emergency Department having been unwell for 5 days with gradually increasing breathlessness and worsening cough, productive of white sputum. Two days earlier he had become confined to bed and was seen by his general practitioner who prescribed antibiotics and prednisolone. However, he continued to deteriorate and this morning was found in bed confused and cyanosed.

His past history includes a 75 pack-year history of smoking with three previous admissions to hospital due to COPD. He has never required ventilatory support nor been admitted to an intensive care unit (ICU). His latest out-patient spirometry, performed 1 month ago, shows a forced expiratory volume of 0.7 l and a forced vital capacity (FVC) of 1.4 l. His current medication consists of inhaled beclomethasone 200 µg bd, inhaled salbutamol as required, amoxycillin 500 mg tds and prednisolone 40 mg daily.

Physical examination reveals a breathless, cyanotic patient using his respiratory accessory muscles. He is drowsy, but easily rousable. He has an irregularly irregular pulse (110 beats.min^{-1}); his blood pressure is 140/85 mmHg. His heart sounds are quiet, but normal, and the jugular venous pressure is not raised. Respiratory rate is 38 breaths.min^{-1} and oxygen saturation measured by pulse oximeter is 82%. Air entry is reduced throughout both lungs, with a widespread, prolonged expiratory wheeze. Examination of other systems is unremarkable.

Arterial blood-gas analysis shows P_aO_2 6.1 kPa, P_aCO_2 9.2 kPa, pH 7.23, HCO_3 36 mmol.l^{-1} and base excess +4.3 mmol.l^{-1}. The patient is receiving 28% oxygen via a venturi mask and nebulised salbutamol and ipratropium is being given. Chest X-ray shows hyperinflated lungs but no focal pathology. Electrocardiogram (ECG) confirms atrial fibrillation but is otherwise normal.

DEFINITION AND DESCRIPTION OF THE PROBLEM

Patients with COPD have expiratory airflow limitation due to chronic bronchitis and/or emphysema. COPD is one of the leading causes of death in the developed world and mortality from this disease has risen dramatically over the past 30 years. In North America and mainland Europe, a larger number of patients with COPD are intubated and ventilated in critical care units compared to the UK. However, recent UK bed expansion, coupled with directives emphasising patient autonomy, are likely to result in significantly greater numbers of such patients receiving ventilatory support. Admissions to ICUs for exacerbations of COPD account for a large proportion of bed-days in North America and mainland Europe, because such patients often require prolonged ventilatory support. COPD is also a common reason for a protracted post-operative ICU admission.

Patients with advanced COPD usually experience periods of clinical stability punctuated by recurrent exacerbations. These exacerbations take the form of acute-on-chronic respiratory failure, characterised by worsening dyspnoea and increasing production of purulent sputum. Many patients also become oedematous during exacerbations after developing 'cor pulmonale'. Most patients admitted with acute-on-chronic respiratory failure will have been previously diagnosed as suffering from COPD. However, a number will present for the first time in established respiratory failure.

PATHOLOGY AND PATHOPHYSIOLOGY OF RESPIRATORY FAILURE IN COPD

The reduction in expiratory airflow in COPD is due to increased airway resistance caused by inflammation, bronchospasm and mucus hypersecretion. In emphysematous patients, loss of parenchymal elastic tissues and surface tension in alveoli results in reduced lung elastic recoil. Forced expiration, while increasing alveolar pressure (and hence driving pressure), also increases dynamic airway compression, resulting in a point of critical closure and no improvement in airflow. As airway obstruction worsens, alveolar emptying is progressively slowed and eventually cannot occur before the next inspiration. This results in incomplete exhalation and the termination of expiration at a point higher than the normal functional residual capacity (FRC). This results in progressive, dynamic hyperinflation of the lung (Figure 3.1).

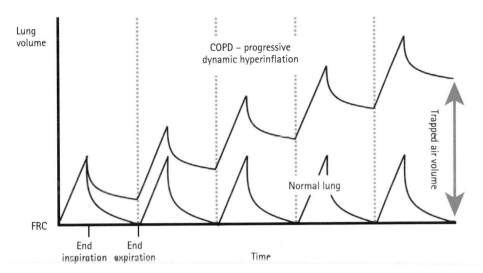

Figure 3.1 – Lung volumes over a period of time in mechanically ventilated patients. In the normal lung, the lung volume returns to FRC at the end expiration. In the COPD patient with airflow obstruction, there is incomplete emptying of the lung with each breath, resulting in dynamic hyperinflation. The volume of trapped air in the lung is illustrated.

Breathing at a higher lung volume increases lung elastic recoil and decreases airway compression, reducing expiratory work of breathing. However, dynamic hyperinflation increases inspiratory work of breathing by two mechanisms. Firstly, both lung and chest wall compliance are reduced at higher lung volumes. Secondly, and of more importance, is the presence of intrinsic positive end-expiratory pressure (PEEPi) which is the residual positive alveolar pressure remaining at the end of expiration. This creates a pressure gradient between the alveolus and the airway beyond the critical closure point (Figure 3.2). A greater inspiratory effort is needed to reverse this pressure gradient. Most COPD patients with acute ventilatory failure have PEEPi values of approximately $10 \, cmH_2O$.

The above pathological changes cause extensive ventilation : perfusion mismatching resulting in hypoxaemia and hypercapnia. Shunting and increased dead space necessitate a higher minute volume in an attempt to maintain normocarbia; this further increases the work of breathing. Respiratory muscles will fatigue when they are no longer able to sustain the mechanical load placed upon them. Once this occurs, respiratory failure develops.

Dynamic hyperinflation also causes the diaphragm and other inspiratory muscles to operate less efficiently due to shorter fibre length and a mechanically disadvantageous position. They are, therefore, poorly able to tolerate the increased mechanical load. Ultimately, a patient with advanced COPD develops intermittent episodes of marked fluid retention associated with raised right heart filling pressures and

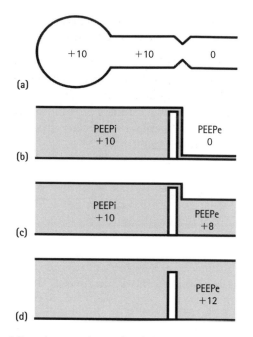

Figure 3.2 – The waterfall analogy can be used to help explain dynamic hyperinflation. Airflow limitation occurs at a point of critical closure (a). Incomplete alveolar emptying results in a build up of pressure – PEEPi. This is analogous to the crest of a waterfall (b). There is a pressure drop across the critical closure point analogous to water falling down the face of the waterfall. The proximal airway pressure at the mouth is represented by water downstream of the waterfall. If this water level rises (c) it will not affect the water level at the crest of the waterfall until it rises higher than the waterfall itself (d). Pressure is measured in cmH_2O.

pulmonary hypertension (cor pulmonale). Its aetiology remains controversial as true right ventricular failure rarely occurs. Both a fall in renal blood flow and endocrine-mediated alterations in salt and water balance contribute to the oedematous state.

Precipitants of acute respiratory failure in COPD

COPD is a progressive illness and will ultimately result in severe disability and death. Patients with advanced disease may present with respiratory failure in the absence of an identifiable precipitant.

Acute pulmonary infections (e.g. acute bronchitis or pneumonia) may occur in up to 75% of COPD exacerbations, partly due to impaired local airway defence mechanisms. Ciliated epithelium is damaged resulting in poor clearance of viscous mucus and bacterial colonisation; around 25% of patients with stable COPD show evidence of tracheobronchial colonisation. During exacerbations, bacteria are present in 50% of patients and viral infections in 10–20%. *Haemophilus influenzae*, *Streptococcus pneumoniae* and *Moraxella catarrhalis* are the most frequent bacterial pathogens. Influenza virus is the commonest viral pathogen encountered. Recently *Chlamydia pneumoniae* has been found in 5–20% of patients.

COPD patients are at a high risk of sputum retention during any acute illness that reduces consciousness (e.g. sepsis) or following surgery. Pneumothoraces are also more common in COPD and may be difficult to distinguish from large bullae in emphysematous patients. Inadvertent placement of a chest drain into a bulla will create a bronchopleural fistula. Patients with COPD are sensitive to the effects of sedative drugs; sedation can precipitate hypoventilation and sputum retention.

THERAPEUTIC GOALS

The therapeutic goals in the management of a patient in respiratory failure due to COPD include:

1. The provision of adequate oxygenation without inducing CO_2 narcosis

2. The reversal of the cause of acute respiratory failure using targeted treatment.

3. The avoidance of invasive mechanical ventilation by the use of non-invasive techniques, where possible.

4. The early recognition of progressive respiratory failure and the need for invasive mechanical ventilatory support.

5. The use of a suitable ventilation strategy.

6. The optimisation of weaning from the ventilator.

7. The provision of an opportunity for survivors of respiratory failure to have a fully informed discussion about their preferences for future critical care support.

THERAPEUTIC OPTIONS BASED ON PHYSIOLOGICAL AND PHARMACOLOGICAL EFFECTS

Assessment of respiratory failure

Arterial blood-gases are likely to show chronic hypercarbia, indicated by an elevated bicarbonate concentration (>30 mmol.l^{-1}) and a base-excess greater than $+4$ mmol.l^{-1}. Renal bicarbonate retention increases serum bicarbonate by 10 mmol.l^{-1} for each 1.3 kPa rise in P_aCO_2 above 5.3 kPa. During acute-on-chronic respiratory failure, further elevation of P_aCO_2 results in an acute respiratory acidosis. The outcome of patients is directly related to the severity of the initial respiratory acidosis. Patients with an initial pH of <7.25 have a significantly greater mortality than those with higher pH recordings.

Spirometry and peak expiratory flow may give an indication of deterioration, if earlier values are available. A chest X-ray is essential to diagnose pneumonia or pneumothoraces, and to rule out other causes of respiratory failure (e.g. pulmonary oedema). In emphysema, the chest X-ray may show bullae (often large) and characteristically hyperinflated lungs with flattened diaphragms. Right ventricular and atrial enlargement, enlarged pulmonary arteries with attenuated distal vessels and oligaemic peripheral lung fields suggest pulmonary hypertension.

The ECG is often normal but may show right ventricular and atrial hypertrophy; there may be right bundle branch block in cor pulmonale. A full blood count may show polycythaemia; an elevated white cell count may be due to infection or corticosteroid therapy. Sputum microscopy and culture are essential in order to identify pathogenic organisms.

Oxygen

The early literature on the treatment of COPD highlighted the potential of uncontrolled oxygen therapy to induce CO_2 retention and narcosis. This led to the universal adoption of controlled oxygen therapy with frequent arterial blood-gases measurements to monitor changes in P_aCO_2. An unfortunate consequence of this literature was the view that oxygen was somehow dangerous and should never be given in an uncontrolled manner. This theory in turn has been discredited and uncontrolled high flow oxygen is once again given to almost all acutely hypoxaemic patients.

This approach can be life saving, but it must be recognised that oxygen can induce CO_2 retention and worsen respiratory acidosis in acute-on-chronic respiratory failure. It is still important to control oxygen therapy in this group. A recent multicentre trial of non-invasive ventilation study in the UK demonstrated that respiratory acidosis will improve in a substantial number of COPD patients simply by substituting controlled for uncontrolled oxygen therapy.

The most appropriate target arterial saturation or P_aO_2 during exacerbations of COPD remains unknown. Traditional (and non-evidence-based) targets of arterial saturations above 90% are probably too high as, even when stable, many COPD patients have arterial saturations well below this level. In the absence of evidence, a target arterial saturation between 85% and 88% is probably adequate, especially if the patient is improving clinically.

Bronchodilators

Nebulised bronchodilators, β_2-adrenergic receptor agonists or anti-cholinergic agents are a standard treatment in acute exacerbations of COPD. However, expiratory airflow limitation is often irreversible in COPD and there is a lack of evidence that either agent is beneficial. Parenteral administration of β_2-adrenergic receptor agonists is possible, but again there is no evidence that they improve outcome.

Intravenous aminophylline is used in COPD. It enhances diaphragmatic contractility and resistance to fatigue *in vitro*, although these effects have not been demonstrated *in vivo*. Most randomised clinical trials have failed to demonstrate any beneficial effect of aminophylline in asthma and two trials of its use in COPD have also been unconvincing. Aminophylline has a narrow therapeutic window and toxicity is common. Numerous drug interactions occur and even in therapeutic doses it is pro-arrhythmogenic. Blood aminophylline levels should be regularly monitored in patients on intravenous therapy.

Corticosteroids

Many patients with acute exacerbations of COPD will receive corticosteroids. In some patients, particularly those with proven reversible airflow obstruction, some improvement in lung function may occur. However, corticosteroids have detrimental catabolic and immunosuppressive effects and these risks should be balanced against their possible benefits.

Antibiotics

Infection is a common precipitant of acute-on-chronic respiratory failure in COPD. Empirical antibiotic treatment is associated with a small but clinically important improvement in peak expiratory flow rate. The choice of antibiotic should follow discussion with local microbiologists. Usually the choice involves an inexpensive broad spectrum antibiotic such as amoxycillin or a second-generation cephalosporin such as cefuroxime.

The incidence of nosocomial pneumonia is high in intubated patients with COPD, due to both the duration of ventilation and the degree of underlying lung impairment. The diagnosis of ventilator associated pneumonia is difficult and the correct choice of antibiotic unclear.

Arrhythmias

Hypoxaemia, hypercarbia, electrolyte disturbance, co-existing ischaemic heart disease, cor pulmonale and drug toxicity promote arrhythmias. Sinus tachycardia, atrial fibrillation or flutter and premature ventricular beats are common in COPD. As would be appropriate in the case described, attention to correcting hypoxia, hypercarbia and electrolyte disturbances is essential before administering anti-arrhythmic drugs. Theophylline compounds should also be stopped if supraventricular tachyarrhythmias occur.

Doxapram

The respiratory stimulant doxapram is often used during hypercapnic episodes of COPD. Few controlled trials of its use exist and evidence for benefit in terms of outcome is at best equivocal. The introduction of non-invasive ventilation to control hypercapnia is likely to significantly reduce the use of doxapram.

Non-invasive ventilation

Non-invasive ventilation is an important recent advance in the management of patients with acute respiratory failure complicating COPD. A number of large, well-conducted, randomised studies have shown that non-invasive ventilation

    (i)   improves survival in COPD patients with an acute respiratory acidosis (pH < 7.35) and

   (ii)   reduces the need for intubation.

The key difference between non-invasive ventilation and conventional mechanical ventilation is the patient – machine interface. A reasonably tight-fitting mask, either nasal or more commonly facial, links the patient to the ventilator. Non-invasive ventilators are often portable, with few alarms, but are functionally equivalent to conventional ventilators in terms of delivery. Non-invasive ventilation and continuous positive airway pressure (CPAP) masks are identical; however non-invasive ventilation and CPAP are not synonymous.

Excluding the interface, non-invasive ventilation and conventional ventilation are identical. The achievement of adequate alveolar ventilation, as indicated by falling P_aCO_2, improving pH and satisfactory inspiratory chest wall movement, is the target. Patients who are likely to improve with non-invasive ventilation will normally show both clinical and biochemical improvement within the first few hours of treatment. A falling respiratory rate, accompanied by improvements in P_aCO_2 and pH, are associated with a good outcome.

Successfully establishing a patient on non-invasive ventilation requires at least as much time and input as conventional ventilation. The service can be physiotherapy-led, nurse-led and medical-led; however, in all cases, the key issue is the availability of trained and competent personnel on a 24-h basis.

Decisions regarding escalation of treatment, if non-invasive ventilation fails, should be made before the start of ventilation. These should involve the patient and, if appropriate, direct family members. Realistic survival prospects and complications should be discussed. A number of patients will decide that non-invasive ventilation should be the limit of their treatment while others will want invasive support, if non-invasive ventilation fails.

The physical location of the non-invasive ventilation service may affect outcome. Most of the randomised controlled trials were conducted in an intensive care environment (Table 3.1).

However, a recent UK multicentre trial demonstrated that non-invasive ventilation can also be successfully used in a general ward setting following training. The

Table 3.1 – Summary of randomised controlled studies in non-invasive ventilation (NIV).

Study	Year	Numbers	Intubations		Hospital mortality	
			Control	NIV	Control	NIV
Bott	1993	60	No data given		30%	10% (NS)
Brochard	1995	85	25%	74%	29%	9%
Kramer	1995	31	31%	73%	13%	6% (NS)
Celikel	1998	30	13% intubated 27% underwent NIV	7%	Intention to treat $n = 15$ Mortality 7%	0% (NS)
Plant	1998	236	27%	15%	20%	10%

Additional references: Bott J, Carroll MP, Conway JH *et al.* Randomised controlled trial of nasal ventilation in acute ventilatory failure due to chronic obstructive airways disease. *Lancet* 1993; 341: 1555–7; Brochard L, Mancebo J, Wysocki M *et al.* Noninvasive ventilation for acute exacerbations of chronic obstructive pulmonary disease. *New England Journal of Medicine* 1995; 333: 817–22; Kramer N, Meyer TJ, Meharg J, Cece RD, Hill NS. Randomized, prospective trial of noninvasive positive pressure ventilation in acute respiratory failure. *American Journal of Respiratory and Critical Care Medicine* 1995; 151: 1799–806; Celikel T, Sungur M, Ceyhan D, Karakurt S. Comparison of noninvasive positive pressure ventilation with standard medical therapy in hypercapnic acute respiratory failure. *Chest* 1998; 114: 1636–42. NS: non-significant.

survival in the treatment group with marked respiratory acidosis (pH < 7.25) was poorer than in some other randomised controlled trials. Consequently, it may be better to initiate non-invasive ventilation in a critical care setting in this group.

Patients who elect to be intubated if non-invasive ventilation fails should also be cared for in a critical care environment. It is important that this group is not allowed to deteriorate on non-invasive ventilation to the extent that a respiratory arrest occurs.

In most cases, non-invasive ventilation is an intermittent method of respiratory support. Support after the first 24 h is gradually reduced depending on arterial gases and clinical status. The indicators for long-term, home non-invasive ventilation in COPD remain uncertain, but a respiratory physician should assess all patients who have received non-invasive ventilation in hospital.

Invasive mechanical ventilation

Indications for mechanical ventilation

Despite attempts to reverse the causes of acute respiratory failure and the use of non-invasive ventilation, some patients will ultimately require intubation and mechanical ventilation. The decision to intubate requires bedside clinical assessment and should not be made solely on the results of arterial blood-gases. Suggested criteria are:

1. A clinical appearance of fatigue and impending respiratory exhaustion.

2. Respiratory rates which remain >36 breaths.min^{-1} despite non-invasive ventilation.

3. Deteriorating level of consciousness due to fatigue and/or hypercarbia.

4. Hypoxia refractory to a high F_iO_2.

5. Inability to protect the airway.

6. Respiratory arrest.

Survival of patients, who progress to respiratory arrest before being intubated, is significantly less than those intubated, once mechanical ventilation is recognised as being unavoidable.

The goals of mechanical ventilation

The objectives of mechanical ventilation in acute respiratory failure complicating COPD are:

1. Correction of blood-gas and acid–base disturbances to normal for the patient.

2. Provision of respiratory support during attempts to reverse the cause of respiratory failure.

3. Reduction in the work of breathing, resting the respiratory muscles and allowing them to recover from fatigue.

4. The use of an appropriate ventilator strategy that avoids dynamic hyper-inflation and facilitates weaning from the ventilator.

Correcting blood-gas and acid–base disturbances

Normocapnia should not be a target in ventilated patients with chronic respira-tory failure, as this group usually has a compensated respiratory acidosis. In the face of chronic hypercarbia there is renal retention of bicarbonate until a steady state is reached at which pH is nearly normal. During acute-on-chronic respiratory fail-ure, further elevation of P_aCO_2 results in an acute respiratory acidosis. This is reflected in this patient's admission arterial blood-gases. Reducing the P_aCO_2 to normal levels would result in an acute respiratory alkalosis. Renal bicarbonate loss would then occur over the following days and, when the patient begins to breathe spontaneously, the P_aCO_2 would return to the original, compensated 'normal' value. An acute respiratory acidosis, which will inhibit weaning, would ensue.

Controlled hypoventilation and permissive hypercapnia are usually well tolerated even at pH levels as low as 7.15–7.20; such hypoventilation reduces the risks of alkalosis and dynamic hyperinflation.

Resting respiratory muscles

The issue of resting fatigued muscles in COPD remains controversial. In healthy volunteers, diaphragmatic fatigue takes over 24 h to resolve; however, resting muscles leads to muscle atrophy. The combination of inactivity, sedative drugs, muscle relaxants and steroids can rapidly lead to loss of muscle mass. In this situation, attempts to rapidly wean patients (possibly onto non-invasive ventilation) may be more effective than 'resting' them on ventilators. In addition, the risk of nosocomial pneumonia increases with duration of invasive ventilation.

Dynamic hyperinflation

A failure of the lung to fully empty at the end of expiration generates a residual alveolar PEEPi. Adding a level of extrinsic PEEP (PEEPe) significantly lower than PEEPi will have no effect. However, because of areas of heterogeneity within the lung, PEEPe that is slightly less than or equal to PEEPi may still increase alveolar pressure.

Complications of dynamic hyperinflation

The adverse effects of PEEPe and PEEPi are identical. The principal haemodynamic action is an acute reduction in venous return to the heart. Pulmonary vessels are also compressed, increasing right ventricular afterload. Subsequent right ventricular dilatation shifts the interventricular septum to the left and reduces left ventricular preload and cardiac output.

Excessive mechanical or hand ventilation, especially immediately after intubation, can worsen dynamic hyperinflation and cause cardiac output and blood pressure to fall; pulseless electrical activity may follow. Disconnection of the patient from the ventilator or breathing circuit will restore venous return by allowing time for complete expiration to occur. Many patients are initially hypovolaemic and will require intravenous fluid to help counteract the effect of positive-pressure ventilation. A few, particularly those with pre-existing left ventricular dysfunction, will also require transient inotropic support.

Barotrauma is common in COPD when the fragile emphysematous parenchyma, often containing large bullae, is over-distended. Pneumothoraces, pneumomediastinum, subcutaneous emphysema and bronchopleural fistulae can all result. Rarely, systemic air embolism or pneumopericardium may occur. Tension pneumothorax is suggested by agitation, tachycardia, tachypnoea, distended neck veins, tracheal shift away from the affected lung and absence of breath sounds with hyper-resonance on the ipsilateral side. Needle thoracocentesis should be performed immediately and can be life saving; this should be followed by placement of a chest drain and the use of measures to reduce dynamic hyperinflation.

Dynamic hyperinflation and PEEPi also have adverse effects on the work of breathing. Both lung and chest wall compliance is reduced at the higher lung volumes seen in dynamic hyperinflation. More importantly, the presence of significant positive alveolar pressure at the end of expiration necessitates a greater inspiratory effort in order to reverse the pressure gradient between the alveoli and the distal airway. PEEPi can, therefore, be seen as a mechanical load that must be overcome in order for the patient to breathe spontaneously or trigger the ventilator. The theoretical concept that applying a level of PEEPe less than PEEPi should prevent dynamic airway closure by 'stenting' open airways and allow lung emptying, remains controversial. As the level of PEEPe approaches that of PEEPi, lung volume actually increases, causing further hyperinflation and subsequent haemodynamic compromise. PEEPe should be applied to a level of about 80% of the measured PEEPi in order to reduce inspiratory work of breathing in the spontaneously breathing or patient-triggered mechanical ventilation.

Detection of dynamic hyperinflation and PEEPi

The existence of PEEPi can be detected in several different ways. These include:

1. Expiratory flow continuing until the onset of the next inspiration can be observed on the graphical display of some ventilators.

2. Observing a delay between the onset of inspiratory effort and the fall in airway pressure at the start of a patient-triggered mechanical breath.

3. Failure of peak airway pressure to change with the application of PEEPe.

However, in order to quantify PEEPi, end-expiratory occlusion must be performed. This is achieved by occluding the expiratory port at end-expiration, allowing equilibration of trapped air in the alveoli with that in the distal airways beyond the critical closing point. The residual positive pressure represents PEEPi, providing the occlusion time is sufficiently long to enable emptying of alveoli with long time constants. Modern ventilators will be able to automatically perform this manoeuvre and display the measured PEEP.

Ventilator management

Ventilator strategies for patients with COPD should use low-tidal volumes, low-minute ventilation and long expiratory times. 'Permissive hypercapnia' should be regarded as the norm. Attempts should be made to wean patients to assisted ventilation modes as quickly as possible. This requires frequent trials of sedation cessation.

Sedation

Patients with acute-on-chronic respiratory failure complicating COPD will usually require sedation and analgesia in order to ensure a reduction in work of breathing, prevent patient-ventilator asynchrony, prevent or limit dynamic hyperinflation, or in severe cases, to limit oxygen consumption and CO_2 production. A number of sedative agents are commonly used. In particular, opiates are useful in suppressing respiratory drive and providing relief from dyspnoea. Benzodiazepines are anxiolytic, hypnotic and may reduce central respiratory drive.

The risks associated with the use of neuromuscular blocking drugs such as prolonged myopathy and thromboembolic disease, mean that paralysis should be reserved for situations where the patient-ventilator asynchrony causes dangerous dynamic hyperinflation. This situation is considerably less common in COPD than in asthma patients.

Bronchodilators

Bronchodilators are standard therapy in the management of the mechanically ventilated COPD patient although there is no good evidence of clinical benefit. Drug delivery is impaired in mechanical ventilation as much of the drug is deposited on the ventilator tubing. Turbulent flow, humidification systems, small tracheal tubes, tidal volumes and inspiratory times also reduce drug delivery.

Weaning from mechanical ventilation

Extubation cannot be contemplated until there has been resolution of the precipitating cause of the exacerbation. The patient must be able to expectorate secretions and protect their airway. Oxygenation should be adequate (on $F_iO_2 < 0.5$ and PEEP <5 cmH$_2$O) and the work of breathing must be balanced by sufficient respiratory muscle strength and endurance.

Reversible causes of respiratory muscle weakness must be sought and treated. Corticosteroids have been shown to cause a myopathy affecting respiratory muscles following prolonged administration. Usually this occurs if doses greater than 30 mg daily are administered for more than 8 weeks; however, this may occur considerably earlier if neuromuscular blocking agents are used concurrently. Muscle weakness can occur due to the use of aminoglycosides, vancomycin, propranolol and quinidine. Malnutrition and electrolyte imbalance (e.g. hypokalaemia, hypocalcaemia and hypophosphataemia) can impair respiratory muscle function. Conversely, overfeeding with excess carbohydrate may increase CO_2 production and the work of breathing. Other causes of respiratory muscle weakness include heart failure, chronic renal failure, diabetes and thyroid dysfunction.

Weaning strategies usually employ T-piece trials or gradual reduction in pressure support ventilation. Neither appears to be more successful than the other; however, the use of synchronised intermittent mandatory ventilation is associated with slower weaning than the other modes. A successful T-piece trial of just 30 min can predict readiness for extubation. Whatever weaning mode is employed, protocol-driven weaning programmes, capable of being executed by nursing or physiotherapy staff, are associated with faster extubation than physician-directed weaning. Non-invasive ventilation has been used in the management of COPD patients with post-extubation respiratory failure with success rates of 83%. Its subsequent use, following planned early extubation in patients has also been successful.

Tracheostomy

The correct timing of tracheostomy in COPD patients is not clear, but it appears to improve patient communication and mobility, allows oral feeding, improves

Table 3.2 – Summary of outcome studies in patients receiving prolonged mechanical ventilation in the intensive care setting.

Study	Year	Number	Duration of mechanical ventilation	Mortality
Seneff	1988–1990	1195	> 7 days	54%
Kurek	1993	6353	All underwent tracheotomy	51%
Gracey	1986–1988	104	29 + days	43%
Spicher	1981–1986	245	10 or greater days	61%
Hill	1993–1995	41	Mean 6 days (1-11.5)	49%

Additional references: Seneff MG, Zimmerman JE, Knaus WA, Wagner DP, Draper EA. Predicting the duration of mechanical ventilation. The importance of disease and patient characteristics. *Chest* 1996; 110: 469–79; Kurek CJ, Dewar D, Lambrinos J, Booth FV, Cohen IL. Clinical and economic outcome of mechanically ventilated patients in New York State during 1993: analysis of 10,473 cases under DRG 475. *Chest* 1998; 114: 214–22; Gracey DR, Naessens JM, Krishan I, Marsh HM. Hospital and post hospital survival in patients mechanically ventilated for more than 29 days. *Chest* 1992; 101: 211–14; Spicher JE, White DP. Outcome and function following prolonged mechanical ventilation. *Archives of Internal Medicine* 1987; 147: 421–5; Hill AT, Hopkinson RB, Stableforth DE. Ventilation in a Birmingham intensive care unit 1993–1995: outcome for patients with chronic obstructive pulmonary disease. *Respiratory Medicine* 1998; 92: 156–61.

pulmonary toilet, reduces the need for sedation and may allow earlier ICU discharge.

USUAL OUTCOME

Hospital mortality for in-patients requiring tracheal intubation and mechanical ventilation with COPD exacerbations is in the region of 50% (Table 3.2).

One-year survival in COPD patients who have been intubated and ventilated varies between 34% and 56%. Quality-of-life surveys of survivors are rare, but one study reported that 53% of survivors were housebound and dependent on carers. In addition, 59% had a worse quality of life compared to before admission. This type of information is important in allowing patients to make informed judgements about their preferences for invasive respiratory support in future exacerbations.

In-hospital mortality in patients receiving non-invasive ventilation was only 10.2% in a multicentre study and 1 year survival was 61.6%.

KEY LEARNING POINTS

1. An increasing number of patients with COPD are likely to be admitted to critical care units in the UK.

2. Non-invasive ventilation reduces the need for intubation and improves survival.

3. Reversible causes of deterioration must be sought and treated.

4. Ventilation strategies should aim to normalise pH and not P_aCO_2.

5. In the intubated patient, mechanical ventilation strategies should aim to minimise dynamic hyperinflation. Low tidal volumes and prolonged expiratory times should be used.

6. Following resolution of the precipitating cause of deterioration, attempts at rapidly weaning from the ventilator should commence. Non-invasive ventilation may be useful as a bridge to complete weaning.

7. Tracheostomy may facilitate quicker discharge from ICU, if rapid weaning fails.

8. Hospital mortality in intubated patients is approximately 50%. In patients treated with non-invasive ventilation it is approximately 10%. One-year survival following intubation is 34–56% but over 60% following non-invasive ventilation.

9. Patients who survive an episode of respiratory failure requiring critical care should be involved in informed discussions about their future preferences for invasive support.

Further reading

1. Sherk PA, Grossman RF. The chronic obstructive pulmonary disease exacerbation. *Clinical Chest Medicine* 2000; **21**: 705–21.

2. Schmidt GA, Hall JB. Acute-on-chronic respiratory failure. In Hall JB, Schmidt GA, Wood LD (eds), *Principles of Critical Care*. New York: McGraw-Hill, 1998: 565–78.

3. Sethi JM, Siegel MD. Mechanical ventilation in chronic obstructive lung disease. *Clinical Chest Medicine* 2000; **21**: 799–818.

4. Plant PK, Owen JL, Elliott MW. Early use of non-invasive ventilation for acute exacerbations of chronic obstructive pulmonary disease on general respiratory wards: a multicentre randomised controlled trial. *Lancet* 2000; **355**: 1931–5.

5. Gladwin MT, Pierson DJ. Mechanical ventilation of the patient with severe chronic obstructive pulmonary disease. *Intensive Care Medicine* 1998; **24**: 898–910.

6. Kress JP, Pohlman AS, O'Connor MF, Hall JB. Daily interruption of sedative infusions in critically ill patients undergoing mechanical ventilation. *New England Journal of Medicine* 2000; **342**: 1471–7.

7. Baudouin S, Blumenthal S, Cooper B *et al.* Non-invasive ventilation in acute respiratory failure. British Thoracic Society Standards of Care Committee. *Thorax* 2002; **57**: 192–211.

4

MIDDLE AGED PATIENT DEVELOPS OLIGURIA AFTER GASTROINTESTINAL HAEMORRHAGE

S Keegan & C Scott

CASE SCENARIO

A previously fit, 55-year-old woman is admitted to hospital after several episodes of melaena and a single haematemesis. Initially, she is noted to have a tachycardia, postural hypotension and has only passed $20\,ml.h^{-1}$ of urine for each of the last 3 h. She is referred to the intensive care unit (ICU) for resuscitation and optimisation prior to investigation and treatment. She has no significant past medical history apart from non-specific hip pain for which she has recently started taking diclofenac sodium 50 mg twice daily.

DEFINITION AND DESCRIPTION OF THE PROBLEM

Acute gastrointestinal haemorrhage is a common cause of ICU admission and is a major cause of morbidity and mortality. In the UK, approximately 5000 deaths per year are directly attributable to upper gastrointestinal haemorrhage. The overall mortality rate in unselected cases is 14%. The elderly are particularly vulnerable, due mainly to their associated co-morbidity. In the majority of cases, the effects of hypovolaemia are responsible for the morbidity and mortality associated with a gastrointestinal haemorrhage. Common symptoms associated with hypovolaemia include pallor, sweating, tachycardia, hypotension, mental confusion and oliguria (defined as a urine output of less than $0.5\,ml.kg^{-1}.h^{-1}$). If resuscitation is not prompt, there is a high risk of end organ damage and multiple organ failure. Therefore, rapid resuscitation of the patient is the primary treatment goal, followed by appropriate treatment of the source of bleeding.

PATHOLOGY AND PATHOPHYSIOLOGY OF THE PROBLEM

Gastrointestinal haemorrhage

The common causes of gastrointestinal haemorrhage and their frequencies are listed in Table 4.1. The majority of cases (85–90%) originate from the upper gastrointestinal tract. Melaena and haematemesis suggest an upper gastrointestinal cause, whilst fresh blood *per rectum* is more typical of the lower gastrointestinal tract.

Mallory–Weiss tears are usually associated with a history of violent or traumatic retching and vomiting, whereas oesophageal varices are associated with the presence of liver cirrhosis. Gastritis and gastric erosions are commonly produced by drugs (e.g. aspirin and non-steroidal anti-inflammatory drugs (NSAIDs)), infections (e.g. cytomegalovirus (CMV)) and excessive alcohol intake. The presence of the urease producing bacterium *Helicobacter pylori* is the most important aetiological factor in the development of peptic ulcers. NSAIDs act by inhibiting cyclo-oxygenase and so reducing prostaglandin synthesis. Prostaglandins inhibit gastric acid secretion and promote mucus secretion, thereby protecting the submucosal layer from acid induced damage. Up to 80% of patients presenting with acute gastrointestinal haemorrhage have recently taken a NSAID. Approximately 20% of patients on long-term NSAID therapy will develop peptic ulcer disease. In addition, NSAIDs inhibit platelet thromboxane production leading to impaired platelet function and a prolonged bleeding time. The presence of hypovolaemic shock and the endoscopic findings suggestive of recent haemorrhage are strong independent predictors of survival.

Table 4.1 – Causes of gastrointestinal haemorrhage.

Upper gastrointestinal bleeding		Lower gastrointestinal bleeding	
Cause	Frequency (%)	Cause	Frequency (%)
Peptic ulcer disease	50	Haemorrhoids	70
Gastric erosions	25	Diverticular disease	10
Gastritis, Duodenitis	10	Angiodysplasia	10
Varices	10	Tumours	6
Mallory–Weiss tear	5	Inflammatory bowel disease	4

Hypovolaemic shock

Blood loss in excess of 15–25% of the circulating volume places the patient at risk of developing hypovolaemic shock. Compensatory sympathetic nervous activity occurs to maintain perfusion of vital organs. The resultant tachycardia and peripheral vasoconstriction is augmented by catecholamine release from the adrenal medulla. Anti-diuretic hormone (ADH) is released from the pituitary gland, increasing water reabsorption in the kidney. Reduced renal perfusion pressure activates the renin–angiotensin system resulting in vasoconstriction and increased aldosterone release causing increased sodium and water retention by the kidney.

However, these compensatory mechanisms may prove inadequate in the presence of severe blood loss. Shock is said to have occurred when each organ's metabolic demand cannot be met because of inadequate tissue perfusion. Anaerobic metabolism increases with the production of lactic acid. The cells swell due to the failure of sodium–potassium pumps and eventually become irreparably damaged. Each organ varies in its ability to withstand hypoperfusion. The kidney becomes compromised sooner because of its high oxygen consumption (approximately 10% of basal whole body oxygen consumption in an organ that represents only 0.5% body weight).

Oliguria and renal failure

The kidneys receive approximately 20% of the cardiac output. The glomerular filtration rate (GFR) is determined by the renal perfusion pressure and the renal vascular resistance. GFR is kept constant by autoregulation of renal blood flow and the tubuloglomerular feedback system. Autoregulation is an intrinsic property of the kidney that relies upon a myogenic response to vary afferent and efferent arteriolar tone. It is effective for mean blood pressures between 70 and 140 mmHg. The tubuloglomerular mechanism varies GFR depending upon the solute load sensed by the macula densa by varying the tone of the afferent arteriole. In addition, locally secreted prostaglandins cause vasodilatation of the afferent arteriole when the renal perfusion pressure is reduced.

As the mean blood pressure falls below approximately 70 mmHg, autoregulation becomes ineffective and GFR becomes directly related to the renal perfusion pressure. Renin acts upon circulating angiotensinogen to cause efferent arteriolar constriction, thereby maintaining an adequate renal perfusion. However, increasing sympathetic stimulation results in vasoconstriction of the renal arteries, further decreasing the renal perfusion pressure and thus GFR. Coupled with the actions of ADH on the renal collecting ducts, the fall in GFR leads to oliguria. With a decrease in the renal perfusion pressure, the parenchymal cells become hypoperfused and eventually hypoxic. The heterogeneous nature of the intra-renal blood flow means the metabolically active cells of the medulla are particularly susceptible to hypoxia. The cells' sodium–potassium pumps fail, causing them to swell and die (i.e. acute tubular necrosis). Inadequately treated hypovolaemia is the most common precipitating factor for acute tubular necrosis. The biochemical differences between pre-renal oliguria and acute tubular necrosis are summarised in Table 4.2.

NSAIDs inhibition of prostaglandin synthesis decreases the kidney's ability to maintain an adequate GFR during periods of hypoperfusion. Rarely, they cause

Table 4.2 – Biochemical features used to differentiate between pre-renal oliguria and acute tubular necrosis.

	Pre-renal oliguria	Acute tubular necrosis
Urine specific gravity	>1.020	1.010–1.020
Urinary osmolality (mosmol.l^{-1})	>500	<350
Urinary sodium (mmol.l^{-1})	<20	>40

direct damage to the kidney by other mechanisms leading to interstitial nephritis and renal papillary necrosis.

THERAPEUTIC GOALS

The therapeutic goals in this patient include:

1. Aggressive resuscitation of the patient using appropriate monitoring and following the principles of A (airway), B (breathing) and C (circulation).

2. Diagnosis and appropriate management of the cause of the gastrointestinal haemorrhage.

3. Instigation of specific renal rescue therapies in an attempt to preserve renal function.

THERAPEUTIC OPTIONS BASED ON PHYSIOLOGICAL AND PHARMACOLOGICAL EFFECTS

Resuscitation of the patient

Airway

The patient should be given a high inspired concentration of oxygen and intubated if her conscious level is reduced due to shock (Glasgow Coma Scale score < 9) or she is at risk of aspiration of blood from the gastrointestinal tract.

Breathing

Tachypnoea is a frequent sign in hypovolaemia. The patient may require ventilatory support if she develops respiratory failure.

Circulation

Venous access should be established using two large bore peripheral cannulae. Blood samples should be sent for immediate crossmatch, haemoglobin, coagulation studies, blood sugar, urea, electrolytes and liver function tests. Initial fluid resuscitation can be with either a synthetic colloid or a crystalloid. With a large gastrointestinal haemorrhage both blood and coagulation products, such as platelets and fresh frozen plasma, will be necessary.

Monitoring

Monitoring should consist of an ECG, pulse oximetry, a urinary catheter, an arterial line and, possibly, a central venous cannula to guide fluid management. In the presence of significant cardiac dysfunction, a pulmonary artery catheter may also prove helpful.

Diagnosis and management of the gastrointestinal haemorrhage

Endoscopy permits precise identification of the bleeding source and aids prognosis, as the risk of rebleeding and death are related to endoscopic findings (Table 4.3). Endoscopy also provides a route for certain therapies.

Table 4.3 – Endoscopic features associated with rebleeding and mortality.

	Probability of rebleed (%)	Mortality (%)
Actively bleeding vessel (spurting or oozing)	85	11
Protuberant vessel in an ulcer bed	33–55	7
Adherent blood clot	22	7
Clean ulcer base	5	2

Large ulcers (>2 cm diameter), and those on either the postero-inferior wall of the duodenal bulb or high in the lesser curvature of the stomach, have an increased risk of rebleeding. In 80% of cases of gastrointestinal haemorrhage due to a non-variceal cause, bleeding ceases spontaneously. However, if a lesion rebleeds, mortality is significantly increased (10–17 fold). Prevention of rebleeding is therefore paramount; treatment options include endoscopic, pharmacological and surgical therapies.

Endoscopic therapies

Endoscopy treatment is the first line method for controlling acute gastrointestinal haemorrhage. It reduces the rate of rebleeding, volume of blood transfused, requirement for surgery and risk of death. Endoscopic methods of treatment include:

1. *Injection.* Although various agents have been advocated, including alcohol, polidocanol, ethanolamine and thrombin, epinephrine (1 : 10 000 alone or in combination with another sclerosant) is most frequently used. The solution is injected around the base of the ulcer. Control may be achieved by tamponade, thrombosis, vasoconstriction or inflammation. Injection has the advantage of being simple, cheap and quick.

2. *Thermal coagulation.* Heat causes tissue oedema, contraction of blood vessels and coagulation of tissue proteins. Endoscopic thermal coagulation makes use of both bipolar electrocoagulation and heater probe

application. Thermal coagulation is sometimes combined with epinephrine injection for the treatment of ulcers that are actively bleeding.

3. *Laser photocoagulation.* A Neodymium : yttrium aluminium garnet (Nd : YAG) or Argon laser can be used to coagulate vessels. Although as effective as other methods, laser coagulation has not gained popularity due to the expense and size of the equipment and the need for specialist training.

4. *Mechanical methods.* Various forms of clips, banding and suturing techniques can be performed endoscopically.

Endoscopic intervention stops bleeding in 80% of actively bleeding ulcers. Of those that rebleed despite therapy, 50% will be controlled with a second treatment.

Pharmacological

1. *H_2-receptor antagonists.* An acidic environment and pepsin secretion impairs platelet function and ulcer healing. However, H_2-receptor antagonists should not be used in isolation in acute gastrointestinal haemorrhage as they do not reduce the immediate risk of rebleeding.

2. *Proton pump inhibitors (PPIs).* The results of some trials suggest that PPIs decrease the risk of rebleeding in patients who do not have active bleeding or an adherent clot at endoscopy. The role of PPIs as a sole agent following an acute gastrointestinal bleed is questionable; however, they are frequently used as an adjunct to endoscopic treatments.

3. *Anti-fibrinolytic agents.* Tranexamic acid does not appear to decrease the incidence of rebleeding.

Vasoconstrictors

Although frequently used in the management of bleeding due to varices, agents such as vasopressin, somatostatin and octreotide have no role in non-variceal bleeding.

Surgery

Endoscopy has significantly reduced the need for surgery for acute gastrointestinal haemorrhage. However, surgery remains the definitive intervention where:

1. endoscopic methods have failed to control bleeding,

2. recurrent bleeding occurs,

3. there is a possibility of the perforation of a viscus, and

4. massive transfusion has been necessary.

Emergency surgery has a high mortality (10–50%). Undersewing of the ulcer is the most frequently performed operation.

Prophylaxis

Once the acute gastrointestinal haemorrhage has been controlled, the patient should be commenced on a regimen to prevent further ulceration. Current recommendations are for a PPI to be combined, where necessary, with antibiotics suitable for *Helicobacter pylori* eradication (see below).

PPIs inhibit the hydrogen–potassium adenosine triphosphatase enzyme system (the proton pump) which is the final step in the production of gastric acid. They decrease acid secretion more effectively than H_2-receptor antagonists. The presence of *Helicobacter pylori* is strongly associated with peptic ulcer disease. If present, eradication therapy should be commenced, as it is associated with improved long term healing rates. Most regimens include a proton pump inhibitor with clarithromycin and either metronidazole or ampicillin. Other prophylactic agents include antacids, sucralfate and misoprostol. Although misoprostol, a synthetic analogue of prostaglandin, may have a specific role in patients taking NSAIDs, it is generally regarded as less effective than PPIs.

Miscellaneous measures

Patients should be encouraged to stop smoking and decrease their alcohol intake.

Oliguria and renal function

In hypovolaemia, the most important factor in preventing pre-renal failure and acute tubular necrosis is the prompt restoration of the intravascular volume and cardiac output. Invasive central venous pressure monitoring may be invaluable in this respect. If oliguria persists after adequate fluid replacement, the following therapeutic interventions may be used:

1. *Vasoconstrictors*. Norepinephrine is frequently used to increase renal perfusion pressure and restore GFR.

2. *Loop diuretics*. Theoretically, loop diuretics (e.g. frusemide) may be of benefit in preventing renal failure, as they increase the resistance of renal tubular cells to periods of ischaemia, by decreasing their metabolic demand and oxygen requirement. The increased diuresis produced by these agents may also reduce the risk of tubular obstruction from cellular debris. However, diuresis may be harmful if it produces hypovolaemia. Frusemide is ototoxic in large doses.

3. *Mannitol*. Mannitol is an inert derivative of the carbohydrate mannose, which acts as an osmotic diuretic. Intravenous mannitol causes water to shift from the intracellular to the intravascular space, thereby decreasing plasma oncotic pressure, blood viscosity and haematocrit. The resultant

increase in plasma volume leads to an increase in the renal arteriolar vasodilator, atrial naturetic factor release. Mannitol may also decrease renal tubular swelling during periods of ischaemia.

4. *Dopamine.* Dopamine is a commonly used and extensively investigated drug for renal rescue in the presence of oliguria. The GFR may be increased through its actions upon dopaminergic (D_1 and D_2), $beta_1$ and alpha-adrenergic receptors. At low doses (1–$3 \, \mu g.kg^{-1}.min^{-1}$) it causes renal vasodilatation (dopaminergic effect). Between 3 and $10 \, \mu g.kg^{-1}.min^{-1}$ dopamine acts as an inotrope via $beta_1$ receptors, causing an increase in cardiac output. Above $10 \, \mu g.kg^{-1}.min^{-1}$, it acts predominantly upon alpha–receptors leading to vasoconstriction and an increase in renal perfusion. Previously, dopamine was thought to act as a diuretic through its inhibition of sodium–potassium ATPase at the renal tubular epithelium. However, now dopamine is now believed to have its renal effects by increased cardiac output alone. Dopamine may actually be harmful. It is known to aggravate gut ischaemia in haemorrhagic shock, induce tachycardia and myocardial ischaemia in hypovolaemia, suppress T-cell proliferation and depress growth hormone secretion in the critically ill. Its use is waning.

5. *Atrial natriuretic peptide analogues.* Atrial natriuretic peptide is naturally secreted by the cardiac atria. It increases renal afferent arteriolar dilatation and efferent vasoconstriction, thus increasing GFR. The related renal natriuretic peptide (urodilatin) has been used in some small trials as a treatment for oliguria. It may improve creatinine clearance, but more studies are needed.

6. *Adenosine antagonists.* Studies suggest that adenosine antagonists, such as theophylline, may prevent acute tubular necrosis caused by radio-contrast dye. However, its routine use is not recommended.

7. *Other drugs.* A multitude of drugs have been investigated as potential renal protective agents. These include endothelin inhibitors, nitric oxide synthatase modulators, insulin-like growth factors, hepatocyte growth factors and epidermal growth factors.

Recommendations

In the presence of hypovolaemia and oliguria, aggressive fluid resuscitation is the only measure that may prevent acute renal failure. None of the drugs above reduces the incidence of renal failure or the need for renal replacement. Nephrotoxic drugs such as NSAIDs, aminoglycosides and angiotensin converting enzyme inhibitors should be avoided.

USUAL OUTCOME

Mortality from acute gastrointestinal haemorrhage depends upon the patient's pre-morbid condition, the cause and the severity of the gastrointestinal bleed. Modern endoscopic techniques have significantly changed the management of such patients. The overall mortality of all unselected cases has remained unchanged over the past 20–30 years, although patient age has steadily risen.

NSAIDs are a major cause of gastrointestinal haemorrhage. It remains to be seen if the new generation of NSAIDs will impact upon this. Mortality from acute renal failure alone remains below 10%. In the presence of multiple organ failure this figure rises to 60−100%.

KEY LEARNING POINTS

1. Gastrointestinal haemorrhage is a common cause for admission to hospital, with NSAIDs being an increasingly common precipitating factor in upper gastrointestinal haemorrhage.

2. Adequate fluid resuscitation is of paramount importance. Central venous monitoring may help guide fluid therapy.

3. Endoscopy is the cornerstone of investigation and management.

4. Low dose dopamine, loop diuretics and mannitol have no place in the treatment of oliguria.

5. Once adequate fluid resuscitation has been completed, vasoconstrictors may have a place if oliguria persists.

Further reading

1. Villanueva C, Blanzo J. A practical guide to the management of bleeding ulcers. *Drugs* 1997; **53**: 389–403.

2. Peterson WL, Cook DJ. Antisecretory therapy for bleeding ulcer. *Journal of the American Medical Association* 1998; **280**: 877–8.

3. Yeomans ND. Approaches to healing and prophylaxis of non-steroidal anti-inflammatory drug associated ulcers. *American Journal of Medicine* 2001; **110**: 24S–28S.

4. Sung JJY. Management of non-steroidal anti-inflammatory drug-related peptic ulcer bleeding. *American Journal of Medicine* 2001; **110**: 29S–32S.

5. Hawkey CJ, Tulassey Z, Szczepanski L *et al.* Randomised controlled trial of *Helicobacter pylori* eradication in patients on non-steroidal anti-inflammatory drugs. *Lancet* 1998; **352**: 1016–21.

6. Dishart MK, Kellum JA. An evaluation of pharmacological strategies for the prevention and treatment of acute renal failure. *Drugs* 2000; **59**: 79–91.

7. Corwin HL. Renal dose dopamine: long on conjecture, short on fact. *Critical Care Medicine* 2000; **28**: 1657–8.

8. Bersten AD, Holt AW. Vasoactive drugs and the importance of renal perfusion pressure. *New Horizons* 1995; **3**: 650–61.

9. New DI, Barton IK. Prevention of acute renal failure. *British Journal of Hospital Medicine* 1996; **55**: 162–6.

10. Oh TE. *Intensive Care Manual.* Oxford: Butterworth-Heinemann, 1997.

5

OLIGURIA AFTER A HIP REPLACEMENT

A E Saayman & G P Findlay

CASE SCENARIO

A 69-year-old male was admitted for an elective hip replacement because of long-standing osteo-arthritis. He is known to have essential hypertension for which he was taking captopril 12.5 mg twice daily. Surgery, performed under a spinal anaesthetic and intravenous sedation, was difficult with significant blood loss. Oral diclofenac (50 mg, thrice daily) was prescribed for post-operative analgesia. Three hours after surgery, the patient developed acute urinary retention, requiring bladder catheterisation. For the next 2 h he appeared to progress well, but continued to lose blood from the surgical drains, causing a persistently low arterial blood pressure (90/60 mmHg). The orthopaedic house officer gave the patient 2000 ml of intravenous crystalloid and then frusemide, 80 mg. Two days after surgery, the patient is oliguric ($\approx 15 \, \text{ml.h}^{-1}$). He is referred to the intensive care team.

DEFINITION AND DESCRIPTION OF THE PROBLEM

Acute renal failure may be defined as a sudden deterioration in the kidneys' ability to excrete metabolic waste products. Creatinine clearance is reduced and the serum urea and creatinine rise. Usually, although not always, urine output falls.

Acute renal failure is common in critically ill patients, with an incidence between 10% and 30%. It occurs less frequently after elective surgery. Acute renal failure is associated with an increased risk of death, especially if associated with sepsis or failure of other organs.

PATHOLOGY AND PATHOPHYSIOLOGY OF ACUTE RENAL FAILURE

The causes of acute renal failure can be divided into pre-renal, renal and post-renal (Table 5.1).

Pre-renal acute renal failure is defined as loss of function in the absence of parenchymal damage and is often secondary to renal hypoperfusion. Common causes include congestive cardiac failure, hypovolaemia or sepsis. Renal causes of acute renal failure include toxins (such as non-steroidal anti-inflammatory drugs (NSAIDs), gentamicin, frusemide and contrast media), glomerulonephritides and other intrinsic renal pathology. Post-renal acute renal failure is caused by obstruction to urine flow and is especially important to recognise as prompt treatment may lead to recovery of renal function at an early stage. Often, the cause of acute renal failure is multifactorial, as in our example, with hypovolaemia, hypotension, obstruction to urine flow and drugs contributing to acute renal failure. If present, pre-existing chronic renal failure will also have an effect.

The pathological processes responsible for intrinsic renal failure are vasoconstriction (in particular, of the afferent arteriole), tubular back-leak and tubular obstruction. Nitric oxide and oxygen free radicals have also been identified as playing a role in ischaemia-induced renal failure.

Obstructive causes of acute renal failure may be classified as congenital (meatal stenosis, ectopic ureters and ureteroceles) or acquired (ureteral strictures, benign prostatic hyperplasia, prostate or bladder tumours, stones, metastatic cancers and

Table 5.1 – Classification of acute renal failure.

Category	Pathophysiological insult	Causes
Pre-renal	Hypovolaemia	Bleeding, vomiting, diarrhoea and burns
	Abnormal fluid distribution	Sepsis and hypoalbuminaemia
	Poor renal blood flow	Congestive cardiac failure and other low cardiac output states
Renal	Nephrotoxins	Drugs, heavy metals, contrast media and myoglobin
	Glomerulonephritides	Primary (membranoproliferative) and secondary (haemolytic ureamic syndrome, eclampsia and scleroderma)
	Intestitial nephritis	Allergic (trimethoprin, β-lactams) radiation and infections (cytomegalovirus and tuberculosis)
	Pyelonephritis	Calculi, strictures and abnormal anatomy
Post-renal	Obstruction to urine flow	Bladder outlet obstruction (cancer) and bilateral upper urinary tract obstruction (papillary necrosis and retroperitoneal fibrosis)

retroperitoneal fibrosis or pregnancy). Alternatively, lesions may be classified into lower-renal-tract lesions (stones), mid-tract lesions (benign prostatic hyperplasia) or upper-tract lesions (ureteral valves and stones). The normal pressure in the renal pelvis is close to zero. The pelvis and calyces dilate with increasing pressure, and the renal papilla becomes ischaemic. Tubules also dilate and increased back pressure results in further functional impairment.

Acute renal failure has several life threatening sequelae. Oliguria may result in fluid overload, leading to pulmonary and generalised oedema. Hyperkalaemia develops as hydrogen ions are excreted in preference to potassium ions; this may cause severe arrhythmias and even cardiac arrest. Hyponatraemia, hypernatraemia, hypercalcaemia, hyperphosphataemia and hypermagnesaemia may also occur. Uraemia itself may cause central nervous dysfunction (drowsiness, stupor and seizures), gastrointestinal bleeding, platelet dysfunction and uraemic pericarditis.

THERAPEUTIC GOALS

The therapeutic goals in this patient include:

1. Early diagnosis of acute renal failure, and the prompt treatment of reversible causes of acute renal failure.

2. General supportive measures.

3. Renal rescue therapies aimed at maintaining urine flow and optimising renal blood flow to alleviate the need for renal replacement therapy.

4. Control of biochemical and metabolic derangement in established acute renal failure by renal replacement therapy.

THERAPEUTIC OPTIONS BASED ON PHYSIOLOGICAL AND PHARMACOLOGICAL EFFECTS

Diagnosis of acute renal failure

The diagnosis and identification of the cause of acute renal failure is usually established by taking a detailed patient history, a physical examination and by undertaking appropriate special investigations. However, it is very important to appreciate that oliguria is usually a surrogate marker of another problem, especially sepsis. The patient's hospital observation charts, notes and old case notes may identify any pre-existing renal dysfunction and provide clues to the current cause of renal failure (e.g. a prolonged period of hypotension following surgery (as in this case) may have been clearly documented in the nursing observation charts).

History

A detailed patient history should include the presenting complaint (e.g. prostatic symptoms may alert the clinician to a post-renal cause of acute renal failure), focused patient questioning, detailed previous medical and surgical history, social history and history of any current medications as well as any known allergies. A family history may reveal a history of polycystic kidney disease.

Examination

Following an assessment of airway, breathing, circulation and disability, a full systematic patient examination is required. The first indication of acute renal failure is usually oliguria. Patients with burns, pancreatitis and those following laparotomy may have large 'third space' fluid losses, leading to acute renal failure. Hypovolaemia is confirmed by the presence of hypotension, tachycardia and cool peripheries. Invasive haemodynamic monitoring to assess pre-load and cardiac output may aid diagnosis. Examination of the abdomen is especially important in the diagnosis of a post-renal cause of acute renal failure, such as an enlarged prostate leading to retention or the presence of a hydronephrotic kidney should prompt treatment of the underlying cause. Hypotension, hypoxaemia, pyrexia and a hyperdynamic circulation may suggest sepsis or the systemic inflammatory response syndrome (SIRS) as the cause of oliguria and renal dysfunction.

Special investigations

Measurement of the serum sodium, potassium, urea and creatinine is essential. There is a progressive rise in serum urea and creatinine concentrations and a rise in serum potassium, especially in the presence of an acidosis. Arterial blood gas analysis is helpful in determining the degree of metabolic acidosis and the degree of respiratory compensation, if the patient is breathing spontaneously. A rapidly rising potassium concentration (>6.0 mmol.l^{-1}), severe metabolic acidosis (base excess > -10 mmol.l^{-1}) and an elevated-serum urea (>50 mmol.l^{-1}) are indications for urgent renal replacement therapy.

Urinalysis is useful in patients with renal failure. Urinary specific gravity is usually greater than 1.020 in pre-renal causes of acute renal failure and closer to 1.010 in patients with intrinsic or post-renal causes. Proteinuria adds to the suspicion of a glomerular injury. Glycosuria, in the absence of hyperglycaemia, suggests a proximal tubular injury. A positive test for blood in the urine suggests an acute glomerular or tubular injury, infection, stones or, possibly, rhabdomyolysis. Intrinsic acute renal failure is often associated with finding urinary sediment. The presence of red cell casts may point to glomerular disease. The presence of eosinophils in the urine suggests a tubulo-interstitial nephritis.

The fractional excretion of sodium in urine may also be helpful. A low value ($<1\%$) in oliguric states suggests a pre-renal syndrome with reabsorption of sodium with functioning renal tubules, whereas values greater than 3% suggest tubular injury. The fractional excretion of sodium is calculated as

$$[Na]_{(urine)} \times [Cr]_{(serum)} / [Na]_{(serum)} \times [Cr]_{(urine)}$$

The serum creatinine clearance is an important measure of renal function. Creatinine clearance is calculated as

$$\text{creatinine clearance (Cl)} = [Cr]_{(urine)} \times \text{urine volume}/[Cr]_{(serum)}$$

The normal value is $120 \, ml.min^{-1}$, and this is similar to glomerular filtration rate in healthy individuals.

Several radiographic investigations are useful in the diagnosis of acute renal failure. Plain abdominal films may show enlarged kidneys, stones or the skeletal changes associated with renal disease. Ultrasound is invaluable in assessing the renal tract and is indicated early in all patients suspected of having acute renal failure. It can reliably identify causes of post-renal acute renal failure (hydronephrosis, full bladder secondary to an enlarged prostate) and provide information regarding kidney size (and presence). Doppler ultrasound can evaluate renal arterial blood flow. Retrograde pyelography can help exclude obstruction. Intravenous pyelography will evaluate renal function and show renal anatomy, although the added nephrotoxicity due to contrast media makes it less popular in current practise.

General supportive measures

The initial management of any critically ill patient focuses on checking the airway, breathing and circulation. In this patient, the airway and respiratory function are satisfactory; however, his circulation requires attention to correct the hypotension.

Renal rescue therapy

Renal rescue therapy is aimed at minimising renal dysfunction and maintaining urine flow. Renal hypoperfusion is often central to the progression of acute renal failure in the critically ill patient, and thus meticulous attention to optimising fluid balance, cardiac output and mean arterial pressure is indicated. Avoiding potential nephrotoxins is also important. Invasive haemodynamic monitoring and appropriate fluid and inotropic therapy may reduce the degree of renal impairment.

Raised intra-abdominal pressure may contribute to deteriorating renal function. Laparotomy and decompression should be considered when the intra-abdominal pressure exceeds $20-25 \, cmH_2O$ as this level is associated with deteriorating renal function. Renal dose dopamine is often used to increase urine flow or to 'prevent' acute renal failure in critically ill patients. However, there is no evidence to support the use of such therapy or any other diuretic. However, diuretics may make fluid balance easier, if urine flow can be maintained.

Renal replacement therapy

Renal replacement therapy has become standard practice in many intensive care units (ICUs). The threshold for renal support may have lowered over the last decade as sophisticated purification systems have become available and staff training and experience has improved.

The indications for renal replacement therapy in the treatment of acute renal failure include salt and water overload, uraemic symptoms, hyperkalaemia and severe acidosis. Renal replacement therapy may also remove water and electrolytes to allow nutritional support or blood product transfusion.

The type of renal replacement therapy used is dependent on the haemodynamic stability of the patient and the locally available renal replacement systems. Stable patients with single organ failure are often managed in specialised renal centres in larger hospitals. The renal replacement therapy of choice in such patients is often intermittent haemodialysis or peritoneal dialysis.

The commonly used techniques for renal replacement therapy in critically ill patients are continuous haemofiltration (arteriovenous or veno–veno haemofiltration) or intermittent haemodialysis. Peritoneal dialysis is now rarely used in the ICU.

Principles of dialysis and haemofiltration

Dialysis removes solutes by passive diffusion across a synthetic semi–permeable membrane. The rate of removal of a substance from plasma is related to solute size and its concentration gradient between plasma and dialysate. The clearance of small molecules such as electrolytes, urea and creatinine is proportional to the permeability of the dialysis membrane, the duration of dialysis and the blood and dialysate flow rates. Clearance of larger molecules is largely related to membrane porosity and dialysis duration and is less dependent on flow rates. Ultrafiltration can be achieved by applying a hydrostatic pressure gradient across the dialysis membrane. The rate of water removal is then dependent on the transmembrane pressure gradient as well as the permeability and surface area of the membrane (Figure 5.1).

Haemofiltration relies on convection of plasma water across a porous membrane and its replacement with a balanced electrolyte solution. Solutes are removed in proportion to their plasma concentration. Membranes may be formed from polysulphone, polyamide or polyacrylonitrile, configured as hollow fibres or parallel plates. Currently, parallel plates are favoured as they have a lower resistance to flow and are associated with greater diffusive clearances of small molecular weight molecules compared to hollow fibre dialysis. Membrane pore size is about 30 000 Da, and so albumin (69 000 Da) is not lost from the circulation. The duration of filtration cycles determines the rate at which uraemia is controlled, while the replacement fluid volume is adjusted to achieve a desired overall fluid balance.

Practical aspects of haemofiltration/haemodialysis

Vascular access

Arteriovenous access has been largely abandoned due to the poor efficacy (secondary to low flow) and complications from arterial access. A temporary double

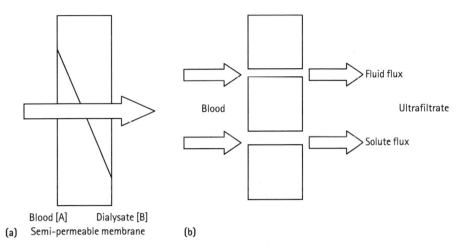

Figure 5.1 – (a) Principle of dialysis: Dialysis relies on the principle of diffusion. A substance moves from a higher concentration [A] in blood to a lower concentration [B] in the dialysate fluid across a semi-permeable membrane. (b) *Principle of haemofiltration:* Solute clearance is by convection and solute drag. Fluid flux is thus an integral part of haemofiltration and a pre-requisite for solute clearance. Fluid replacement (either pre- or post-filter) is required to ensure normovolaemia.

lumen catheter made of polyurethane (which is semi-rigid and usually used for shorter periods of renal support) or silicone (a more flexible material for longer periods of central venous cannulation) is placed aseptically in the internal jugular, subclavian or femoral veins. The choice of vessel varies between centres, but the femoral route is usually preferred in patients with coagulation abnormalities and those who cannot be positioned in the Trendelenburg position. The length, diameter, elasticity, number and position of distal holes all play a role in the efficacy of the catheters. Central venous catheter related bacteraemia is a well-recognised problem in critically ill patients and meticulous attention to catheter care is necessary. Catheters should be changed if the site becomes inflamed, or the patient develops a bacteraemia or an increase in infective markers such as temperature, raised white cell count or a raised C-reactive protein levels.

Anticoagulation

The coagulation cascade is activated as soon as blood comes into contact with the extra-corporeal circuit. Anticoagulation is required to extend filter life, improve filtration fraction and clearance characteristics. Many critically ill patients have abnormal coagulation characteristics, but anticoagulation is usually required for all but those with very deranged clotting function. Several anticoagulation regimes are currently used; these include unfractionated heparin (systemically or into the arterial limb of the filter), prostacyclin and low-molecular weight heparin.

The combination of heparin ($200-400\,u.h^{-1}$) into the arterial limb of the filter with systemically administered prostacyclin ($2.5-5\,ng.kg^{-1}.min^{-1}$) may limit platelet aggregation, extend filter life and function and reduce the risk of bleeding (Figure 5.2).

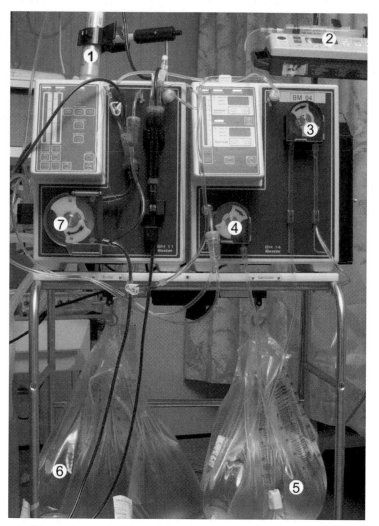

1. Filter unit (containing filter membrane)
2. Anticoagulation pump
3. Replacement fluid pump
4. Filtrate pump
5. Replacement fluid
6. Effluent fluid
7. Blood pump

Figure 5.2 – A haemofilter machine.

Replacement fluid

The ultrafiltrate produced during haemofiltration is replaced by an appropriate volume of electrolyte solution to achieve the desired fluid balance. Replacement solutions contain physiological concentrations of sodium, chloride, calcium and magnesium. Depending on their plasma concentrations, potassium and phosphate may be added. In addition, a buffer (usually lactate) is also administered, as bicarbonate is lost across the membrane. However, lactate may cause myocardial depression and liver dysfunction may impair the metabolism of lactate into bicarbonate. Furthermore, the exogenous administration of lactate invalidates serum lactate as a marker of tissue perfusion. An alternative is to use bicarbonate as the buffer; however, it cannot be pre-mixed in replacement solutions due to precipitation and bubbling. Therefore, sodium bicarbonate is often administered separately when lactate-free replacement solutions are used. Although there are these theoretical advantages to avoiding lactate as a buffer, there does not appear to be any clinical advantage. Trace elements such as copper, selenium and zinc are not routinely added to replacement fluids, and their levels should be closely monitored.

Drug handling and dosage adjustments

Principles of extra-corporeal drug removal

Several physiochemical and pharmacokinetic characteristics of drugs affect their removal by dialysis or haemofiltration, including molecular weight, volume of distribution, protein binding, inter-compartmental rate constants and fraction eliminated by the kidneys. Molecular size is an important factor in drug removal by conventional haemodialysis, but less so during continuous haemofiltration as the membranes used resemble those used in high-flux dialysis. Drugs with a molecular weight less than 500 Da are easily removed by conventional haemodialysis, whereas those drugs with a molecular weight between 500 and 1000 Da are more effectively cleared by haemofiltration. Drugs with a large volume of distribution are mainly tissue bound with only a small intravascular fraction; intermittent techniques are less effective than continuous renal replacement techniques for these drugs. Drugs that are highly protein bound are poorly cleared by continuous techniques, as the drug–protein complex is too large to filter. The filtration of the unbound fraction of drug depends on physiochemical factors such as pH, relative concentrations of drug and protein, bilirubin concentration, heparin therapy, concentration of free fatty acids and the presence of other agents which may compete for drug binding sites, particularly on proteins. The contribution of renal clearance to total body clearance of a drug will also affect drug dosing. Thus, if a drug is excreted unchanged by the kidney, its clearance will be severely reduced in acute renal failure. The total body clearance of the drug will then dramatically increase with renal replacement therapy. If a drug is not primarily excreted by the kidney, its clearance may not be extensively augmented by renal replacement therapy.

Impact of filter membranes on drug removal

The clearance of solutes using the same filtration technique, but different filter membranes, may yield different results. Other filter characteristics that affect clearance include surface area and the ultrafiltration constant. The sieving coefficient, which is the ratio of drug concentration in the ultrafiltrate to that in the pre–filter plasma water, is an index of the drug's ability to traverse the filter membrane. Sieving coefficients near unity implies that a drug has relatively free passage across a membrane. For example, the sieving coefficient for ampicillin is 0.69, while that for ceftazidime is 0.9, reflecting ceftazidime's easier passage across the filter.

Individualisation of drug therapy for patients on renal replacement therapies

It is important to consider the type of renal replacement therapy and filter, rate of ultrafiltraton and blood flow, as they will affect drug dosage regimes. Blood and ultrafiltrate sampling can be used to estimate drug disposition during filtration or dialysis. Drug clearance can then be estimated and standard pharmacokinetic dosage equations can be used to adjust drug dosages.

Complications of renal replacement therapy

It is important to be aware that, despite the apparent ease of use of current renal replacement therapy techniques, they are potentially extremely dangerous therapies. Potential problems include the following.

Vascular access problems

The necessity for large bore double–lumen vascular access for renal replacement therapy may expose the patient to all the complications of central venous cannulation including bleeding, pneumothorax, arterial or nerve injury, air embolus and catheter related infection.

Bleeding

This is usually due to systemic anticoagulation. Upper gastrointestinal bleeding can be a major problem as gastric erosions are more likely in the critically ill uraemic patient.

Hypotension

This is a major problem, especially during haemodialysis. The aetiology of hypotension during renal replacement therapy is multifactorial and involves pre–existing cardiovascular instability, hypovolaemia secondary to ultrafiltration, autonomic dysfunction, hypo–osmolality and the accumulation of lactate or acetate.

Dysequilibrium syndrome

This is caused by hypo–osmolality and may lead to headache, nausea and restlessness in awake patients. Seizures may occur secondary to cerebral oedema.

The syndrome tends to develop in moderately uraemic patients who are receiving brisk haemodialysis and is caused by water influx into the brain.

Hypoxaemia

This tends to occur during the first 2 h of dialysis. This may be caused by hypo-ventilation (because carbon dioxide diffuses into the dialysate) and leucocyte aggregate micro-emboli.

Vitamin deficiency

Water-soluble vitamins are easily filtered and need to be replaced with trace elements, as long as renal replacement therapy is in progress.

Hypophosphataemia

Hypophosphataemia is common in any critical illness and may be exacerbated with acute renal failure.

Lactate accumulation and acidosis

Lactate used as a buffer agent may accumulate if the liver is unable to metabolise the lactate load to bicarbonate. This can lead to hyperlactaemia. At the same time, acidosis will develop due to the loss of bicarbonate in ultrafiltrate, if it is not replaced by lactate conversion.

Errors in fluid and electrolyte balance

Large volumes of ultrafiltrate are produced and replacement fluid administered over a 24-h period. Small discrepancies in matching input/output can lead to large errors in desired fluid balance. Fortunately modern renal replacement therapy machines are much more reliable and have minimised this problem.

Technical problems

Problems include those associated with the disconnection of the extra-corporeal circuit (e.g. air entrainment and blood loss).

USUAL OUTCOME

Acute renal failure carries a high mortality. With modern supportive techniques, patients should not die of electrolyte or metabolic disturbance as a consequence of acute renal failure. However, the mortality from single organ renal failure remains around 10–20%, but this is increased to at least 60% if there are three or more concurrent organ system failures. In patients who do recover, tubular lesions usually heal completely, and there is usually ($\approx$97%) no obvious residual renal impairment in the long term.

KEY LEARNING POINTS

1. Acute renal failure is a common problem in critically ill patients. If its recognition and treatment is delayed, death may occur due to hyperkalaemia and cardiac arrythmias.

2. Renal failure is classified into pre-renal, renal and post-renal causes. In practice, renal failure in critically ill patients is often due to several different aetiologies.

3. A careful history, chart review and clinical examination will often point to the cause of acute renal failure and highlight reversible factors.

4. Renal rescue therapy, using 'renal dose' dopamine or diuretics, has no place in the management of incipient or established acute renal failure.

5. In critically ill patients, continuous veno–veno haemofiltration is the method of choice to treat the electrolyte, metabolic and fluid balance derangements of acute renal failure. Despite the apparent simplicity of modern technology, it must be remembered that this is a potentially dangerous form of therapy.

6. Acute renal failure carries a high mortality in critically ill patients. The mortality rate increases with additional organ failures to reach at least 60%, when three organ systems have failed.

7. Despite this high mortality, renal function will recover in a matter of weeks in survivors, and there is usually no residual renal impairment.

Further reading

1. De Mendonca A, Vincent JL, Suter PM *et al.* Acute renal failure in the ICU: risk factors and outcome evaluated by the SOFA score. *Intensive Care Medicine* 2000; **26**: 915–21.

2. Groeneveld AB, Tran DD, Van der Meulen J *et al.* Acute renal failure in the medical intensive care unit: predisposing, complicating factors and outcome. *Nephron* 1991; **59**: 602–10.

3. Scwilk B, Wiedeck H, Stein B *et al.* Epidemiology of acute renal failure and outcome of haemodiafiltration in intensive care. *Intensive Care Medicine* 1997; **23**: 1204–11.

4. Brivet FG, Kleinknecht DJ, Loiret P *et al.* Acute renal failure in intensive care units – causes, outcome, and prognostic factors of hospital mortality: a prospective, multicenter study. *Critical Care Medicine* 1996; **24**: 192–8.

5. O'Leary M, Bihari D. Preventing renal failure in the critically ill. *British Medical Journal* 2001; **322**: 1437–8.

6. ANZICS Clinical Trials Group. Low dose dopamine in patients with early renal dysfunction: a placebo-controlled randomised trial. *Lancet* 2000; **356**: 2139–43.

7. Meyer M. Renal replacement therapies. *Critical Care Clinics* 2000; **16**: 29–58.

8. Joy M, Matske G, Armstrong D *et al.* A primer on continuous renal replacement therapy for critically ill patients. *Annals of Pharmacotherapy* 1998; **32**: 362–74.

6

ADVERSE DRUG REACTION FOLLOWING CORONARY ANGIOGRAPHY

C Waldmann

CASE SCENARIO

A 47-year-old businessman, who smoked 20 cigarettes per day, developed a mild rash and pruritis immediately after the intravenous injection of Iohexol during coronary angiography. He has a past history of penicillin allergy. Following intravenous administration of hydrocortisone (100 mg) and chlorpheniramine (10 mg), the itchiness improved. Angiography proceeded and demonstrated good left-ventricular function, but 80% stenosis of the mid-left anterior descending coronary artery. Angioplasty was successfully performed on this lesion.

About 1 h later, the patient developed a swollen face and periorbital oedema. Within 20 min, his breathing became laboured and wheezes were apparent. He developed hypotension with an arterial blood pressure of 85/40 mmHg, and a sinus tachycardia of 130 beats.min^{-1}. He was admitted to the intensive care unit (ICU).

After consultation with the immunology department, a blood sample was taken for serum tryptase level 1 h after arrival in ICU. The measured level was reported as 28 ng.ml^{-1} (normal: 2–14 ng.ml^{-1}).

DEFINITION AND DESCRIPTION OF THE PROBLEM

This patient developed an acute reaction to the iodine-containing contrast media used during the coronary arteriography. Adverse reactions to drugs can be classified as predictable or unpredictable. Predictable reactions are usually dose dependent, reproducible, and are often accepted as expected side effects of the drug (e.g. hypotension, following administration of thiopentone). Unpredictable drug reactions may be classified as anaphylactoid or anaphylactic and are dose independent. Parenteral exposure, especially via the intravenous route, tends to result in a fast and severe reaction. Most severe reactions occur almost immediately after exposure to the triggering agent; but in some instances, symptoms may not appear until 3–4 days after exposure. Common causes of anaphylaxis include penicillin, latex, radiocontrast media and insect bites or stings. An interesting aspect of anaphylaxis is that not all sensitised individuals will react when re-exposed to the antigen; it has been estimated that 10–20% will react with penicillin, 20–40% with radiocontrast media and 40–60% with insect bites or stings (Table 6.1).

Table 6.1 – Incidence of anaphylaxis to commonly used drugs.

Drug	Incidence of reactions (%)	Number at risk
Food	0.0004	1099
Penicillin	0.7–10	1.9–27.2 million
Radiocontrast media	0.22–1	22 000–100 000
Latex	0.0001	220
Insect stings	0.5–5	1.36–13.6 million
Total		3.29–40.9 million

Modified from Neuget AI, Ghatak AT, Miller RL. Anaphylaxis in the United States; an investigation into its epidemiology. *Archives of Internal Medicine* 2001; 161: 15–21.

The other common cause of anaphylaxis in hospital patients is anaesthetic agents. In a survey in France between 1997 and 1999, a network of 38 French allergo-anaesthesia clinics (Groupe d'Etudes des Reàctions Anaphylactoides Peranes-thésiques) reported on anaphylaxis during anaesthesia. A total of 467 anaphylactic incidents were referred to the network of which 69% were due to muscle relaxants, 12% due to latex, 8% were due to antibiotics (penicillin 22, cephalsporins 11, vancomycin 2, rifampicin 1 and quinolone 3), thiopentone was responsible for 1% and propofol for 2% of the reactions. Colloids were responsible for 5% of the reactions (gelofusin and hetastarch).

Anaphylaxis is only one of the complications of angiography and other complications need to be excluded (Table 6.2).

The molecular similarity between penicillins and cephalosporins leads to cross-sensitivity, although the exact incidence of cross-sensitivity may be lower than the 10% that is often quoted. Data also suggest that individuals with penicillin allergy may be allergic to many other drugs, including contrast media, thereby implying a state of general immune hyper-responsiveness. Importantly, patients may react to penicillins, even if there has been no previous exposure. Reactions to iodine-containing contrast media occur in up to 10% of exposures, but are usually

Table 6.2 – Common complications of coronary angiography.

Complications	Incidence (%)
Major	
Death	0.1–0.2
Myocardial infarct	0.1–0.3
Cerebrovascular accident	0.1–0.3
Transient	
Vasovagal collapse	1.5–2.5
Access problems	1–3
Arrhythmias	0.3–0.5
Allergy	<2
Infection	<0.5
Nephropathy	<0.5

Modified from Adair OV, Havranek EP. *Cardiology Secrets.* Philadelphia: Hanley and Belfus, 1994: 51

Table 6.3 – Incidence of clinical features of anaphylaxis or anaphylactoid reactions (%).

Cardiovascular collapse	88
Bronchospasm	36
Facial and periorbital oedema	24
Generalised oedema	7
Rash	13
Erythema	45
Urticaria	8.5

Modified from The Association of Anaesthetists of Great Britain and Ireland. Guidelines for the Management of Anaphylaxis (www.aagbi.org/pdf/Anaphyld.pdf).

mild. However, approximately 1–3% of patients who receive contrast are at risk of a severe reaction. Pre-treatment with antihistamines and/or steroids, and the use of low molecular weight contrast media, decreases the incidence of allergic reactions.

The clinical manifestations of contrast allergy may be delayed for 6 h and, in 5% of patients, recur up to 72 h after the initial exposure (biphasic reaction). The main features of a severe allergic reaction include flushing of the skin, swelling of the skin and mucous membranes, bronchospasm and hypotension. Cardiac arrest and multiple organ failure may follow severe reactions (Table 6.3).

PATHOLOGY AND PATHOPHYSIOLOGY OF ALLERGIC REACTIONS

Historically, the first report of anaphylaxis was described in hieroglyphics of 2640 BC, when an Egyptian pharaoh died after a wasp sting. The term 'anaphylaxis' is

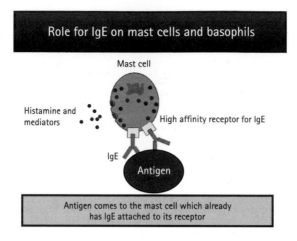

Figure 6.1 – Interaction of IgE with mast cells leading to vasoactive mediator release. Reproduced with permission of Prof. H. Waldmann, William Dunn School of Pathology, Oxford, UK.

derived from the Greek 'ana' meaning backward and 'phylaxis' meaning protection. Classically, anaphylactic reactions occur after exposure to a foreign protein (antigen) that stimulates the production of IgE antibodies (Type I reaction). After the initial exposure, antibody levels fall, but IgE binds to mast cells and basophils. If there is a further exposure to the antigen, the antigen binds with IgE antibodies and results in the release of mediators, including histamine, slow-reacting substance-A (SRS-A), leukotrienes, tryptase and prostaglandins. These substances increase mucous secretion, bronchial smooth muscle tone and vascular permeability, causing airway oedema, bronchospasm and hypotension (Figure 6.1).

Anaphylactoid reactions are clinically indistinguishable from anaphylactic ones, but they neither involve IgE nor prior exposure to the antigen. The underlying mechanisms include the release of vasoactive substances (e.g. histamine), direct histamine release from mast cells or complement activation by either the classical or alternative pathways. Anaphylactoid reactions are the usual process by which contrast media cause allergy. Treatment for both anaphylactic and anaphylactoid reactions is similar. When mast cells and basophils degranulate, serum tryptase is elevated for few hours. Therefore, measurement of serum tryptase levels is helpful in the diagnosis of anaphylactic and anaphylactoid reactions.

Contrast media are commonly used for radiological procedures in cardiology and urology, but allergic responses, which are usually minor, occur in 3–12% of patients. Iodine is used to provide radio-opacity and is the only element satisfactory for intravascular radiological contrast studies. The other constituents of the contrast media act as carriers for the iodine, increasing its solubility, while reducing its toxicity. A multicentre study in 1990 in Japan covering 337 647 subjects demonstrated an incidence of 3.13% (0.04% serious) for non-ionic contrast media compared to

12.66% (0.22% serious) for ionic contrast media. While most reactions appear within 30 min with ionic preparations, delays of several hours may be apparent following the administration of non-ionic preparations.

The major disadvantage of conventional ionic contrast media, such as hypaque, is their extremely high osmolality. However, they are cheaper than the non-ionic contrast media. Non-ionic contrast media (e.g. ioxaglic acid) have a lower osmolality and cause less discomfort, fewer adverse reactions (3.13% versus 12.66%) and fewer life-threatening reactions (0.04% versus 0.22%) compared to the ionic formulation. Reactions to ionic contrast media may be related to their hyperosmolality causing:

1. erythrocyte damage;

2. endothelial damage, including damage to the blood–brain barrier;

3. systemic vasodilation, leading to hypotension caused by rapid intra-vascular volume expansion, and the blood volume may be increased by 20% within a few minutes;

4. myocardial depression and myocardial ischaemia.

Other proposed mechanisms for reaction to contrast media include the inhibition of enzymes such as cholinesterase resulting in an increased concentration of acetyl-choline, causing vagal stimulation.

THERAPEUTIC GOALS

Once an adverse reaction has occurred, the therapeutic goals include:

1. The termination of the reaction, using adrenaline.

2. The prevention of airway obstruction, using tracheal intubation and, if required, tracheostomy.

3. The adminstration of oxygen.

4. The reversal of brochospasm, using adrenaline and conventional bronchodilators.

5. The reversal of hypotension, using patient positioning, intravenous fluids and adrenaline.

THERAPEUTIC OPTIONS BASED ON THE PHYSIOLOGICAL AND PATHOPHYSIOLOGICAL EFFECTS

Prevention

If possible, every effort should be made to prevent an allergic reaction occurring. In general, this means taking a thorough drug history from the patient and exploring any potential drug reactions in detail. If true anaphylaxis is likely and the cause is known, the precipitating antigen should not be administered. Pre-treatment with intravenous corticosteroids, H_1- and H_2-receptor antagonists is sensible.

Recognition

Following the injection of any agent, flushing and swelling of the skin and mucous membranes, bronchospasm and hypotension should alert the medical attendants to the possibility of an anaphylactic reaction.

Immediate action

If anaphylaxis is suspected, an immediate action drill should be started. Every clinician should practice such a drill, if their clinical practice involves the administration of drugs or agents likely to lead to anaphylaxis (Table 6.4).

Table 6.4 – Cockpit drill for managing severe allergic reactions.

Stop administration of the antigen or remove the patient from contact with it.
Secure the airway.
Administer 100% oxygen.
Secure intravenous access.
   Administer adrenaline 0.5–1.0 mg; repeat at 5-min intervals depending on the response.
   Adrenaline may be given intramuscularly, as this is safer outside of an ICU.
Set up an adrenaline infusion.
Commence an intravenous infusion (avoid colloids that have a higher incidence of allergy).
Administer 10 mg chlorpheniramine intravenously.
The use of H_2-receptor antagonists remain unproven, but intravenous ranitidine, 50 mg, is usually administered.
Administer intravenous hydrocortisone 100 mg.

The following recommendations are also made:

1. Do not use contrast media in isolated clinical setting.

2. Never leave the patient unattended.

3. Ensure patent intravenous access.

4. If there is a past history of allergy, use non-ionic contrast media and pre-treat the patient with corticosteroids.

5. Ensure that full resuscitation facilities are available.

6. Ensure that all staff have up-to-date cardiopulmonary resuscitation training.

7. Tag the notes and X-rays of all patients who have experienced a prior drug reaction.

Observation and organ support

All patients who suffer a serious allergic reaction should be managed or observed on a critical care area, so that they can be closely observed for a biphasic response. Severe reactions, which do not respond quickly to therapeutic measures of the immediate action drill will require the full range of organ support available on ICU.

Investigation of the allergy

Investigation of allergic drug reactions should be conducted in consultation with a Clinical Immunologist/Allergy Specialist. However, during the crisis, efforts should be directed to ensuring an adequate airway, breathing and circulation, as no tests have an immediate management benefit. Once patient stability is achieved, a full blood count and differential white cell count should be performed. Blood should be taken for the measurement of complement levels 3, 6, 12 and 24 h after the reaction. Immunoglobulin electrophoresis should also be performed. After 1 h of the reaction, a sample of 10 ml of venous blood should be taken, the serum separated and stored at −20°C before being sent to a reference laboratory for the measurement of serum tryptase levels. In addition, urine samples should be collected at 2 and 24 h for the measurement of methylhistamine. These samples should be sent to the National Adverse Drug Reactions Advisory Service in Sheffield for radioallergosorbent antibody testing (RAST) or radioimmunoassay (RIA) testing. A full description of the patient's symptoms, drugs given and the timing of the reaction should be provided. All adverse reactions should be reported to the Committee on Safety of Medicines.

Skin prick tests, which test the presence of sensitised lymphocytes, are used to investigate patients who have had an anaphylactic reaction. However, it may be difficult to confirm the precipitating agent, as patients are often exposed to several agents simultaneously. During skin prick testing, it is usual to use a diluted drug. If no wheal, flare or pruritis occurs within 15 min, the test is negative for the agent studied. Some centres then use an intradermal injection, but this itself may be associated with anaphylaxis. A positive skin prick test is limited in value. Up to 90% of patients who are positive for penicillin allergy are actually able to tolerate the drug.

USUAL OUTCOME

Allergy is one of the more common reactions that occur during coronary angiography. Usually, it results in a mild skin rash, itching or tremor and responds well to intravenous hydrocortisone and chlorpheniramine. Death is very rare; with timely and appropriate intervention, patients usually improve rapidly.

KEY LEARNING POINTS

1. Allergic drug reactions may be predictable or unpredictable. Unpredictable reactions result from anaphylactic or anaphylactoid reactions.

2. The main features of severe allergic reactions include flushing of the skin, swelling of the skin and mucous membranes, bronchospasm, decreased cardiac output and hypotension. Cardiac arrest and multiple organ failure may follow severe reactions.

3. A history of hayfever, asthma or pencillin allergy in a patient aged between 20 and 50 years old, increases the probability of reactions to contrast media, especially if ionic media are being used.

4. The emergency treatment of anaphylactic or anaphylactoid reactions involves the administration of adrenaline, oxygen, fluids, antihistamines and corticosteroids.

5. All severe reactions should be followed up by a clinician specialised in allergy.

Further reading

1. Bochner BS, Lichtenstein LM. Anaphylaxis. *New England Journal of Medicine* 1991; **324**: 1785–90.

2. Wasserman SI, Marquardt DL. Anaphylaxis. In Middleton E, Reed CE, Ellis EF *et al.* (eds), *Allergy: Principles and Practice.* St Louis: CV Mosby, 1988: 1365–76.

3. Sidhu PS, Dawson P. *Guidelines for the Management of Reactions to Intravenous Contrast Media.* London: Royal College of Radiologists, 1993.

4. The Association of Anaesthetists of Great Britain and Ireland. *Guidelines for the Management of Anaphylaxis* (www.aagbi.org/pdf/Anaphyld.pdf).

5. Palmer FG. The RACR survey of intravenous contrast media reactions. Final report. *Australasian Radiology* 1988; **32**: 621–8.

6. Almén T. The etiology of contrast medium reactions. *Investigative Radiology* 1994; **29**: 537–45.

7. Schwartz LB, Metcalfe DD, Ottesen EA. Tryptase levels as an indicator of mast cell activation in systemic anaphylaxis and mastocytosis. *New England Journal of Medicine* 1987; **316**: 1622–66.

8. Katayama H, Yamaguchi K, Kozuka T *et al.* Adverse reactions to ionic and non-ionic contrast media: a report from the Japanese Committee on the safety of contrast media. *Radiology* 1990; **175**: 621–8.

9. Fisher MM, Baldo BA. Anaphylactoid reactions during anaesthesia. *Recent Advances in Anaesthesia and Analgesia* 1994; **18**: 159–78.

10. Kagy L, Blaiss MS. Anaphylaxis in children. *Pediatric Annals* 1998; **27**: 727–34.

7

SEPSIS AND MULTIPLE ORGAN FAILURE FOLLOWING AN EMERGENCY LAPAROTOMY

D Watson & G Wray

CASE SCENARIO

A 70-year-old male patient with diverticular disease and rheumatoid arthritis, for which he normally takes oral prednisolone (10 mg daily), is admitted to the intensive care unit (ICU) following an emergency laparotomy. At surgery, faecal peritonitis and an inflammatory mass in the left iliac fossa are found; a defunctioning colostomy is fashioned. The patient is transferred to the ICU for post-operative care. An epidural catheter has not been placed. Within 2 h of arriving in the ICU, the patient's arterial blood pressure falls to 80/45 mmHg and his urine output diminishes to 20 ml.h^{-1}.

DEFINITION AND DESCRIPTION OF THE PROBLEM

Peritonitis places this patient at high risk of developing the systemic inflammatory response syndrome (SIRS), sepsis and their sequelae including multiple organ dysfunction syndrome (MODS) or multiple organ failure (MOF) (Tables 7.1 and 7.2). The definitions of these conditions are precise but there is often overlap between them or a progression from one to another.

Elderly patients with significant co-morbidities commonly present for emergency surgery and have a high post-operative mortality rate. Complicating issues for this patient include rheumatoid arthritis (e.g. restrictive neck movements, atlanto-axial subluxation, fibrotic lung disease and joint pain). Adrenal suppression, due to long-term steroid therapy increases the risk of infection, produces glucose intolerance and delays post-operative healing.

Table 7.1 – The definition of SIRS.

The SIRS is defined as two or more of the following:
- Temperature >38°C or <36°C
- Heart rate >90 beats.min^{-1}
- Respiratory rate >20 breaths.min^{-1} or P_aCO_2 < 4.3 kPa
- White cell count >12 × 10^9 l^{-1}, <4 × 10^9 l^{-1} or >10% immature forms on peripheral blood film

Sepsis
- SIRS plus a documented infection

Severe sepsis
- Sepsis plus organ dysfunction (Table 7.2), hypoperfusion or hypotension
- Hypotension defined as systolic arterial blood pressure <90 mmHg or a reduction of >40 mmHg from baseline in the absence of other causes for hypotension (e.g. cardiogenic shock)

Septic shock
- Severe sepsis plus persisting hypotension despite adequate fluid resuscitation

Modified from Consensus Conference Definitions of SIRS, sepsis and septic shock. American College of Chest Physicians/ Society of Critical Care Medicine Consensus Conference: Definitions for sepsis and organ failure and guidelines for the use of innovative therapies in sepsis. *Critical Care Medicine* 1992; 20: 864–74.

Table 7.2 – Typical manifestations of multiple organ dysfunction.

Acute deterioration in mental state not due to sedation or primary underlying disease of the central nervous system

Acute hypoxaemic respiratory failure defined by a P_aO_2/F_iO_2 ratio less than 40 kPa (300 mmHg) in the absence of primary underlying pulmonary disease

Acute renal failure defined by either oliguria (a urine output of <0.5 ml.kg^{-1}.min^{-1} for at least two consecutive hours) or a rise in serum creatinine concentration ≥177 μmol.l^{-1} within the previous 48 h in the absence of primary underlying renal disease

Acute hepatic failure defined by at least two of the following in the absence of primary underlying hepatic disease:
- serum bilirubin >43 μmol.l^{-1}
- serum alanine transaminase concentration greater than twice the upper limit of the normal range
- prothrombin time >1.5 times the control value or an International Normalised Ratio >1.5 in the absence of systemic anticoagulation

Thrombocytopaenia defined by either a platelet count <75 ×10^9 l^{-1} or an acute decrease (i.e. ≥50%) within the previous 24 h in the absence of primary underlying disease of the bone marrow

Disseminated intravascular coagulation defined by at least two of the following:
- thrombocytopaenia or
- prothrombin time >1.5 times the control value or an International Normalised ratio >1.5 in the absence of systemic anticoagulation
- d-dimer titre >0.5 μg.ml^{-1} or fibrin split product titre >10 μg.ml^{-1}

A plasma lactate >2 mmol.l^{-1} or a base deficit >−5 mmol.l^{-1}

PHYSIOLOGY AND PATHOPHYSIOLOGY OF SEPSIS AND SIRS

Following injury the body normally mounts an inflammatory response in an attempt to neutralise invading micro-organisms. This response includes the activation of inflammatory cells such as macrophages, release of pro-inflammatory cytokines and activation of the coagulation and complement systems. Acute phase proteins, arachidonic acid metabolites, nitric oxide and reactive oxygen species (ROS) are also produced. Some of these mediators have direct effects, for instance nitric oxide can be bactericidal, whereas others (e.g. interleukin (IL) 6) stimulate B lymphocytes to produce antibodies and T-cells to proliferate. Mostly, the body's response to a given insult is appropriate and balanced; along with the many pro-inflammatory mediators released there are also anti-inflammatory mediators that prevent an uncontrolled systemic reaction. Classically, patients with SIRS, sepsis or septic shock are thought to have an overwhelmingly large response to a given insult. The trigger event leading to SIRS may include surgery, trauma, burns, pancreatitis and sepsis. Following the trigger, a chain of events ensues, normally starting with the release of tumour necrosis factor alpha (TNFα), IL-1 and many other mediators. This is often termed the cytokine cascade (Figure 7.1).

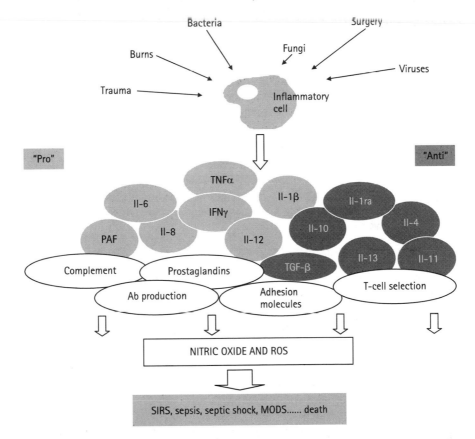

Figure 7.1 – A variety of stimuli leading to the release of the cytokine cascade and other media-tors. Pro-inflammatory cytokines are shown in light grey, anti-inflammatory in dark grey. Ab: antibody; ROS: reactive oxygen species, for example, peroxynitrite.

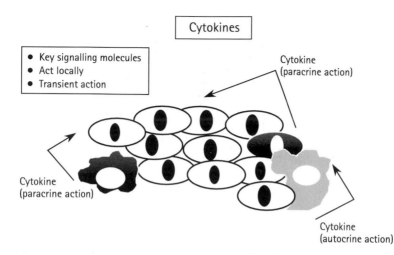

Figure 7.2 – Cytokines released from inflammatory cells can act in an autocrine (acting on self) or paracrine (acting on neighbouring cells) fashion.

Cytokines are low molecular weight (<80 kDa) proteins that regulate the amplitude and duration of the immune response. They are key signalling molecules and include the interleukins, growth factors, chemokines and interferons (Figure 7.2).

Patients who are immunocompromised may not be able to mount an adequate inflammatory response. These patients may have a predominant compensatory anti-inflammatory response syndrome (CARS) and high concentrations of anti-inflammatory cytokines (Figures 7.1 and 7.3).

Consequently, patients mounting an overwhelming response, and those who under respond, may fare equally badly.

The clinical manifestations of severe sepsis include haemodynamic changes, capillary leakage and later organ dysfunction. The haemodynamic changes invariably include hypotension, due mainly to vasodilation caused by nitric oxide, bradykinin, prostaglandins and other vasoactive mediators, but there is also fluid loss through leaky capillaries. Patients usually have an increased cardiac output with a low systemic vascular resistance and often appear warm with peripheral vascular dilatation. However, if the patient is concurrently hypovolaemic or has a fixed low cardiac output, patients will often have cold peripheries and appear 'shut down'. Previously, the terms 'warm shock' and 'cold shock' have been used to describe these two clinical states. However, these terms are misleading and unhelpful, as they imply different disease processes rather than the variants of the same condition. When the effects of sepsis are severe, organ dysfunction or failure may occur. The following organ dysfunctions are common: acute renal failure, acute lung injury

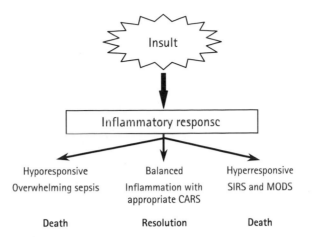

Figure 7.3 – The inflammatory response to a given insult may be balanced, hypo- or hyper-responsive. Patients falling into the latter two categories have a higher mortality. Compensatory anti-inflammatory response syndrome (CARS), systemic inflammatory response syndrome (SIRS) and multi-organ dysfunction syndrome (MODS). (Reproduced from Bellingan G, Inflammatory cell activation in sepsis. *British Medical Bulletin* 1999; **55**: 12–29 by permission of Oxford University Press.)

(ALI) or acute respiratory distress syndrome (ARDS), hepatic failure and haematological failure (e.g. thrombocytopaenia or disseminated intravascular coagulation (DIC)) (Table 7.3).

For this patient, there is another consideration; the effects that long-term steroid therapy have on the stress response to surgery. Normally, the tissue injury, pain and hypovolaemia associated with trauma or surgery initiate a neuroendocrine reflex that leads to a release of adrenocorticotrophic hormone (ACTH) from the anterior pituitary. ACTH stimulates the adrenal cortex to release glucocorticoids (mainly cortisol) and mineralocorticoids (aldosterone). Cortisol has many metabolic actions; it stimulates the conversion of protein to glucose (catabolic action), enhances the storage of glucose as glycogen and antagonises insulin promoting gluconeogenesis and hence raising blood glucose. Cortisol also facilitates the actions of catecholamines, decreases vascular permeability and suppresses synthesis of prostaglandins and leucotrienes. These actions will have the effect of maintaining blood pressure and blood volume. Furthermore, aldosterone increases reabsorption of sodium from the distal convoluted tubules and collecting ducts, and hence reduces urine output. Patients on long-term steroid therapy have a blunted pituitary–adrenal axis and are unable to mount a glucocorticoid response. Therefore, this patient is at increased risk of cardiovascular collapse, hypoglycaemia or hyponatraemia, if exogenous steroids are not administered.

Table 7.3 – Criteria for patients at high risk of developing serious complications after surgery.

Previous severe cardiorespiratory illness (e.g. chronic obstructive pulmonary disease restricting daily
  activity; chronic heart failure New York Heart Association [NYHA] class III–IV)
Extensive ablative surgery planned for carcinoma or prolonged surgery of >8 h (e.g. total gastrectomy,
  radical pancreaticoduodenectomy, total colectomy)
Severe multiple trauma (e.g. more than three affected organs; or two or more systems; or two or more
  body cavities opened)
Massive acute blood loss (e.g. >8 units; blood volume <1.5 l.m^{-2}; haematocrit <0.2)
Age >70 years and evidence of limited physiologic reserve in one or more vital organs (e.g. liver,
  elevated bilirubin; kidney, elevated creatinine; heart, NYHA II to IV; lungs, dyspnoea after walking on
  level ground)
Shock (i.e. mean arterial pressure <60 mmHg; urinary output <20 ml.h^{-1})
Septic shock (i.e. positive blood culture or septic focus; white cell count >13 × 10^9 l^{-1}; spiking fever
  to 38.8°C for 48 h; mean arterial pressure <70 mmHg)
Respiratory failure (i.e. P_aO_2/F_iO_2 ratio <200; P_aO_2 <60 mmHg on fraction of inspired oxygen >0.4;
  mechanical ventilation required for >48 h)
Acute abdominal catastrophe with haemodynamic instability (e.g. pancreatitis; gangrenous bowel;
  peritonitis; perforated viscus, including traumatic causes; gastrointestinal bleeding)
Acute renal failure (i.e. creatinine >200 μmol.l^{-1})
Acute hepatic failure (e.g. bilirubin >51 μmol.l^{-1}; albumin < 30 g.l^{-1}; lactic
  dehydrogenase >200 units.l^{-1}; alkaline phosphatase >100 units.l^{-1}; ammonia >70 μmol.l^{-1})
Late state vascular disease involving aortic disease
Severe nutritional problems (e.g. weight loss >10 kg in past 6 months; plasma albumin <30 g.l^{-1};
  osmolality <280 mmol.l^{-1})

Modified from Tukala J, Meier-Hellmann A, Eddleston J *et al.* Effect of dopexamine on outcome after major abdominal
surgery. A prospective randomized multicentre study. *Critical Care Medicine* 2000; **28**: 3417–23.

THERAPEUTIC GOALS

For this patient, most therapy is supportive, as few specific treatments exist that
directly reverse the effects of sepsis and so alter outcome. Supportive therapy is
aimed at maintaining:

1. Tissue oxygenation, preventing hypoxaemia by oxygen therapy and
    supporting ventilation.

2. Cardiovascular stability by optimum fluid balance.

3. Normothermia.

4. Adequate analgesia in conjunction with anxiolysis.

5. End–organ function.

Specific therapy might include:

1. Appropriate antibiotic cover.

2. Peri–operative steroid cover (e.g. intravenous hydrocortisone).

3. Tight control of blood sugar.

Survival after surgery is dependent, in part, on adequate cardiac reserve. Some practitioners believe that the peri-operative course can be improved by optimising circulating blood volume and cardiac function by achieving targets for cardiac output, oxygen delivery and oxygen consumption. The targets that have been used in many studies of both surgical and critically ill patients were originally defined in the 1980s and are known as 'Shoemaker's' goals. These were originally chosen as they appeared to represent 'survivor values' when high risk surgical patients were studied retrospectively. They are

1. cardiac index (CI) $>4.5\,l.min^{-1}.m^{-2}$;

2. oxygen delivery (DO_2) $>600\,ml.min^{-1}.m^{-2}$;

3. oxygen consumption (VO_2) $>170\,ml.min^{-1}.m^{-2}$.

There is some evidence of benefit in optimising patients undergoing high risk surgery to achieve some of these goals in the peri-operative period and targeting mixed venous oxygen saturation in the early stages of sepsis. However, there are considerable risks in using large doses of inotropes to achieve Shoemaker's goals in patients who fail to respond to simpler treatment or are in the late stages of septic shock. Post-operatively, if optimal filling is achieved and perfusion pressure is optimal, the use of inotropes, aimed at anything other than normal haemodynamics for the patient concerned, does not seem appropriate.

THERAPEUTIC OPTIONS BASED ON PHYSIOLOGICAL AND PHARMACOLOGICAL EFFECTS

Immediate care

The first priority in the post-operative period is maintenance of an adequate airway and ventilation using sedation (e.g. midazolam and parenteral analgesics). If the patient is hypothermic, active warming should be started using warmed fluids, warmed humidified inspired gases and warm-air devices (e.g. Bair hugger®).

Cardiovascular support

Intravenous fluids should be given to achieve an optimal filling pressure and cardiac output using a Frank–Starling curve for the individual. The effects of fluid administration on peripheral and central temperature, urine output, haemodynamics, oxygen transport and lactate levels should be monitored. The choice of fluid used in resuscitation has undergone considerable scrutiny in recent years. Most intensive care specialists would opt for the use of colloids (e.g. gelatin or starch solutions) in the hope that they will remain in the circulation longer. Recently, the use of human albumin solution has declined. The haemoglobin should be kept above $8\,g.dl^{-1}$ in all patients except those with ischaemic heart disease where a level $>10\,g.dl^{-1}$ is recommended.

If hypotension persists, or there is evidence of organ hypoperfusion (e.g. lactic acidosis or oliguria), more aggressive haemodynamic support is required. Under these circumstances enhanced haemodynamic monitoring (e.g. pulmonary artery catheter, oesophageal Doppler or pulse contour analysis monitor (PiCCO®)) is indicated. At all times, the first priority is to ensure that the circulating volume is adequate prior to starting or increasing inotropic or vasopressor support. Careful monitoring of pulmonary artery occlusion pressures is particularly important in a patient who has signs of pulmonary oedema, ALI or ARDS. If haemodynamic monitoring confirms that the patient is vasodilated with a high cardiac output, vasopressors should be used to restore mean arterial pressure to at least 80 mmHg or to near the patient's normal blood pressure. Norepinephrine $(0.05–2\,\mu g.kg^{-1}.min^{-1})$ is often the agent of choice in these circumstances. Whatever agent is chosen, the systemic vascular resistance index should not be allowed to rise above 1500 dynes.$s^{-1}.cm^{-5}$.

If the CI is low, dobutamine $2.5–25\,\mu g.kg^{-1}.min^{-1}$ should be used to maintain the CI between 2.5 and $3.5\,l.min^{-1}.m^{-2}$. Alternative agents include dopamine $(2.5–20\,\mu g.kg^{-1}.min^{-1})$ or epinephrine $(0.01–2\,\mu g.kg^{-1}.min^{-1})$. More recently dopexamine and enoximone have been used to treat septic patients. It should be noted that these agents, like dobutamine, are potent vasodilators and usually need to be used in conjunction with a vasopressor agent to maintain blood pressure. In some cases, shock may become refractory to treatment, with escalating doses of norepinephrine being required. This is due, in part, to receptor down-regulation and may respond to steroid administration. Relative steroid deficiency can be confirmed by a short synacthen test, but may be difficult to interpret in this patient. Where receptor down-regulation is thought likely, an alternative vasopressor agent may be needed. Following the withdrawal of angiotensin and the failure of the nitric oxide synthase inhibitor, laevo-N-monomethyl-L-arginine (L-NMMA) in clinical trials, choice is limited. Vasopressin and terlipressin have been used, but neither has been studied in a randomised controlled study for their effectiveness in treating septic shock.

If cardiovascular support is effective, sequential lactate levels should fall and there will be improvement in the markers of tissue perfusion (e.g. warm peripheries, urine output $>0.5\,ml.kg^{-1}.min^{-1}$).

Steroids and other specific therapies

For many years, high dose corticosteroids were used in the management of shock. However, large doses of methyl prednisolone (e.g. $30\,mg.kg^{-1}$) do not improve outcome in severe sepsis or septic shock even when administered within a few hours of diagnosis. However, there is more recent evidence that the use of smaller, more physiological doses of steroids are beneficial. In the patient described, steroids should be administered pre-operatively (e.g. hydrocortisone 100 mg intravenously) and continued post-operatively (e.g. hydrocortisone infusion $1–2\,mg.h^{-1}$) until recovery is complete. Other novel therapies tried in sepsis or septic shock include the use of monoclonal antibodies directed against endotoxin, various cytokines or their receptors; none of these can be recommended at present. Currently, there is considerable interest in the naturally occurring cytokine antagonists, mediators of coagulation (e.g. activated protein C), intensive insulin therapy and the role of genetic susceptibility to systemic inflammation. It has been shown that tight glycaemic control (i.e. blood sugar regulated between 4.1 and 6.1 mmol.l^{-1}) can significantly reduce morbidity, mortality and the number of episodes of sepsis in critically ill surgical patients.

Surgical debridement

The importance of surgical drainage or removal of the source of any infection cannot be overemphasised. Regular sepsis screening may identify secondary infective or inflammatory episodes, which require investigation to identify treatable causes (e.g. abscess formation, pancreatitis, acalculous cholecystitis). The routine replacement of monitoring lines is not necessary; however, if routine surveillance cultures reveal line related sepsis or there is evidence of a new septic episode without an obvious source, changing intravascular lines is indicated.

Multiple organ failure

Although patients similar to ours are frequently admitted to the ICU for a short period of 'warming, waking and weaning', they sometimes fail to stabilise and develop post-operative pyrexia, hypotension and persistent acidaemia. Post-operative chest X-rays to confirm central venous line placement and tracheal tube position may also reveal diffuse pulmonary infiltrates consistent with ALI.

It is currently impossible to identify those individual patients who will progress to MOF. However in this patient, the operative findings of extensive faecal peritonitis together with an early hypotensive episode, increase the chances of post-operative complications. Early significant hypoalbuminaemia, unexpected hypoglycaemia, early leucopenia (i.e. $<4000 \times 10^9 \, l^{-1}$) and large ongoing fluid requirements with underlying coagulopathy suggests impending MODS.

This patient is at particular risk of developing intra-abdominal distension secondary to ileus or fluid sequestration; raised intra-abdominal pressures may create an abdominal compartment syndrome. This is identified by raised intravesical pressures (commonly >30 mmHg) and worsening renal function. A laparostomy may be needed to decompress the abdomen and may improve urine output and renal function. The bowel has been termed the 'engine of multiple organ failure'. Enteric gram-negative organisms or their endotoxins may leak continually from hypoperfused bowel into the circulation (i.e. bacterial translocation), where they then amplify the initial inflammatory signal or cause secondary insults. Early enteral nutrition (nasogastric or nasojejunal tube feeding) is thought to reduce the chances of bacterial translocation by stimulating gut perfusion.

Haemodynamic dysfunction (Chapter 1), respiratory support for severe hypoxaemia (Chapter 2) and management of oliguric renal failure (Chapter 4) and hepatic dysfunction (Chapter 9) are dealt with elsewhere. When sequential organ dysfunction occurs, hypotension, hypoxaemia, acidosis will exacerbate the clinical situation, thereby impeding recovery. Patients who have a long stay on ICU complicated by MODS often also develop peripheral neurological failure (e.g. critical illness neuropathy). This leads to profound weakness which can lengthen hospital stay even further, thus placing the patient at risk from further nosocomial infection and other hazards (e.g. pulmonary embolism).

USUAL OUTCOME

High risk surgical patients who achieve Shoemaker's goals for haemodynamic and oxygen transport values within the first 24 h after surgery do well. In contrast, those patients with severe sepsis who fail to stabilise quickly are most likely to have a protracted post-operative course. In elderly patients, failure of three organs, 1 week after emergency abdominal surgery, is associated with significant (>50%) mortality. Even when recovery occurs, prolonged in-patient stay can be anticipated.

For those patients with ongoing organ failure and escalating vasopressor or inotropic support, the prognosis is bleak. In patients developing vasoplegia or unresponsive vasodilatation, vasopressin infusion may prove transiently effective while strategies to intensify organ support are revisited. Some patients suffering sepsis complicated by coagulopathy and requiring high dose vasopressor support may develop early signs of bilateral symmetrical digital ischaemia, which can lead to gangrene. In such circumstances, discussions with family will need to focus on the overwhelming nature of the disease process and the futility of resuscitative measures if cardiorespiratory arrest occurs. The comfort and dignity of such critically ill but dying patients can then be planned with the multidisciplinary team.

KEY LEARNING POINTS

1. Survival following surgery is dependent on adequate cardiac reserve. Elderly patients with coexisting disease have a high peri-operative mortality of up to 30%.

2. Pre-emptive therapy with fluid and inotropes to increase oxygen transport before elective or emergency surgery has been associated with improved survival. Some experts advocate wide application of such strategies in high risk surgical patients.

3. For patients with established critical illness (e.g. post-operative sepsis), prompt intervention may help prevent deterioration to MOF and improve outcome. Delays in treatment are likely to be associated with the development of refractory tissue hypoxia. Adequate volume replacement and restoration of blood pressure to pre-morbid values with maintenance of cardiac output to within the normal range are essential in the peri-operative period.

4. Those patients with established septic shock usually require enhanced haemodynamic monitoring (e.g. pulmonary artery catheter, oesophageal Doppler).

5. Surgical drainage to remove infected tissue or pus is essential.

6. A stable first post-operative day helps differentiate those who can respond with only moderate support and those patients who are likely to have a protracted post-operative course.

7. MOF is a problem greater than the sum of its individual parts and will generally only improve if the patients recover from their primary pathology.

8. Adjunctive or prophylactic therapies are at present of unproven value. Activated protein C may be of help, in patients with the highest probability of death it is contraindicated where risk of haemorrhage exists.

Further reading

1. Shoemaker WC, Appel PL, Kram HB *et al*. Prospective trial of supranormal values for survivors as therapeutic goals in high-risk surgical patients. *Chest* 1988; **94**: 1176–86.

2. Wilson J, Woods I, Fawcett J *et al*. Reducing the risk of major elective surgery: randomised control trial of preoperative optimisation of oxygen delivery. *British Medical Journal* 1999; **318**: 1099–103.

3. Rivers E, Nguyen B, Havstatd S *et al*. Early goal-directed therapy in the treatment of severe sepsis and septic shock. *New England Journal of Medicine* 2001; **345**: 1368–77.

4. Cochrane Injuries Group Albumin Reviewers. Human albumin administration in critically ill patients: systemic review of randomised controlled trials. *British Medical Journal* 1998; **317**: 235–40.

5. Hebert PC, Wells G, Blajchman MA *et al.* A multicenter, randomised, controlled clinical trial of transfusion requirements in critical care. *New England Journal of Medicine* 1999; **340**: 409–17.

6. Task Force of the American College of Critical Care Medicine. Practice parameters for haemodynamic support of sepsis in adult patients in sepsis. *Critical Care Medicine* 1999; **27**: 639–60.

7. Levy B, Nace L, Bolleart PE *et al.* Comparison of systemic and regional effects of dobutamine and dopexamine in norepinephrine-treated septic shock. *Intensive Care Medicine* 1999; **25**: 942–8.

8. Annane D. Effects of the combination of hydrocortisone (HC) and fludrocortisone (FC) on mortality in septic shock. *Critical Care Medicine* 2000; **28**: A46 (Abstract 63).

9. Bernard GR, Vincent JL, Laterre PF *et al.* Recombinant human protein C Worldwide Evaluation in Severe Sepsis (PROWESS) study group. Efficacy and safety of recombinant human activated protein C for severe sepsis. *New England Journal of Medicine* 2001; **344**: 699–709.

10. Van den Berghe G, Wouters P, Weekers F *et al.* Intensive insulin therapy in critically ill patients. *New England Journal of Medicine* 2001; **345**: 1359–67.

8

POST-OPERATIVE PNEUMONIA AND FLUID LOSSES

G Morgan

CASE SCENARIO

A 63-year-old man has deteriorated acutely 5 days after resection of an annular carcinoma of the ascending colon. An epidural for intra- and post-operative analgesia had been sited but was removed after 48 h and patient controlled analgesia with morphine substituted. He had been requiring intensive physiotherapy for the previous 3 days but today his peripheral arterial oxygen saturation is 85% on 40% oxygen. He is drowsy and confused and unable to co-operate with physiotherapy; he persistently removes his oxygen mask. His temperature is 38.5°C. He is maintaining his airway and his trachea is central. He is tachypnoeic (22 breaths.min^{-1}), and is both centrally and peripherally cyanosed. His pulse rate is 110 beats.min^{-1} but is regular and bounding. His arterial blood pressure is 100/60 mmHg. Capillary-refill time is less than 3 s. His abdomen is slightly distended and diffusely tender. He has produced 1500 ml of green coloured naso-gastric aspirate over the previous 24 h. He is oliguric, producing only 200 ml of urine in the last 12 h. A chest X-ray shows bilateral basal collapse and a small pleural effusion on the right. A decubitus abdominal radiograph shows gaseous distension throughout the small bowel with fluid levels.

At his pre-operative assessment he weighed 90 kg and was 168 cm tall, giving a body mass index of 32 kg.m^{-2}. He smoked 15 cigarettes per day between the ages of 20 and 55, stopping because he was becoming increasingly breathless on exertion. He is now breathless on one flight of stairs. In the wintertime, he has a persistent productive cough with mucoid sputum and a tendency to contract respiratory tract infections. He is prescribed beclomethasone and salbutamol inhalers on a regular basis.

Pre-operative ventilatory function tests showed severe airflow limitation due to chronic obstructive pulmonary disease (COPD); his forced expiratory volume in 1 s (FEV_1) to forced vital capacity (FVC) ratio was 55%. Now arterial blood gas analysis shows a mixed respiratory and metabolic acidaemia (pH 7.25, P_aCO_2 7.5 kPa, P_aO_2 9 kPa, HCO_3^- 30 mmol.l^{-1}, F_iO_2 0.4, base excess -12 mmol.l^{-1}). His current blood tests are haemoglobin concentration 16.8 g.dl^{-1}, white blood cell count 18×10^9 l^{-1}, Na^+ 128 mmol.l^{-1}, K^+ 3.2 mmol.l^{-1}, Cl^- 92 mmol.l^{-1}, HCO_3^- 30 mmol.l^{-1}, urea 30 mmol.l^{-1} and creatinine 220 μmol.l^{-1}.

DEFINITION AND DESCRIPTION OF THE PROBLEMS

This patient has two main problems, namely deteriorating pulmonary function on a background of COPD, and fluid and electrolyte losses from the gastrointestinal tract secondary to bowel dysfunction.

Even in healthy subjects, ventilatory function gradually deteriorates with age. This is reflected in an increased alveolar–arterial oxygen tension difference $(D(A - a)O_2)$ from a minimum of 2 kPa (15 mmHg) in young adults to 5 kPa (37.5 mmHg) in the elderly. Normal values of P_aO_2 are around 9.5 kPa in subjects aged over 60 years when breathing air. Advanced age is associated with greater ventilation/perfusion (V/Q) inequalities, which increase further with anaesthesia. Loss of tissue elasticity results in a decrease in functional residual capacity (FRC) below closing capacity (i.e. the lung volume at which airway closure occurs). Additional peri-operative factors exacerbating the deterioration in ventilatory function include opiate and neuromuscular blocking agents, volatile anaesthetic agents, pain, abdominal distension and immobility. In the immediate post-operative period the residual effects of anaesthetic agents and narcotics are a major influence. Falls in FRC are worst on the second post-operative day and are greatest in patients having surgery near the diaphragm. Effort dependent ventilatory function tests (i.e. FVC, FEV_1, and peak expiratory flow rate (PEFR)) deteriorate over the first 48 h following abdominal surgery. Episodes of sleep apnoea are common in patients who have received opiates. Alterations in diaphragmatic function also contribute.

Gastrointestinal motility invariably ceases temporarily following abdominal surgery. The incidence of post-operative nausea and vomiting following abdominal surgery may be as high as 40%. Ileus is defined as a reversible decrease in gut motility secondary to a physiological derangement and resulting in functional obstruction to the passage of bowel contents. After abdominal surgery the stomach (3 days) and colon (5 days) are slower to recover normal motility than the small bowel (5–10 h). In critically ill patients, ileus is a more common problem than obstruction and tends to resolve in a predictable manner within 5 days. During this period, ileus can have significant effect on fluid management because of naso-gastric losses and sequestration within the bowel lumen.

PATHOLOGY AND PATHOPHYSIOLOGY OF THE PROBLEMS

COPD is the progressive development of chronic bronchitis and emphysema and is usually associated with long-term exposure to tobacco smoke and atmospheric pollution. The disease is characterised by progressive airflow limitation with an accelerated age-related decrease in FEV_1. Chronic inflammation of the bronchial epithelium of large and small airways leads to hypertrophy and hyperplasia of mucous glands within the bronchial walls and an increase in the number of goblet cells in the lining epithelium at the expense of ciliated cells. Excessive production of mucus causes bronchial and bronchiolar obstruction; there may also be second-ary colonisation of the usually sterile terminal bronchioles with pathogenic organisms such as *Haemophilus influenzae* and *Streptococcus pneumoniae*. Emphysema results from destruction of inter-alveolar septa and enlargement of the air spaces distal to the terminal bronchioles. Both V and Q are reduced in affected areas. The loss of elastic tissue contained in the inter-alveolar septa contributes to the closure of small airways particularly during expiration resulting in air trapping. Hyperinflation of the lung causes flattening of the diaphragm so rendering it inefficient in drawing air into the thorax. Progressive destruction of the pulmonary vasculature and hypoxic pulmonary vasoconstriction leads to pulmonary hypertension and eventually right ventricular failure. Chronic retention of carbon dioxide should be suspected if the plasma bicarbonate is greater than $30\,mmol.l^{-1}$.

Anaesthesia and surgery are associated with areas of atelectasis that are demonstrable on CT scan. General anaesthesia impairs mucociliary transport causing atelectasis and sputum retention and so predisposing to post-operative respiratory infection, especially in patients whose ventilatory function is compromised by pre-existing disease. In the immediate post-operative period, opiates, inadequate pain relief and immobility also contribute to the development of atelectasis. No single test accurately predicts the development of ventilatory failure after abdominal surgery but poor ventilatory function is associated with smoking, COPD, poor general health, prolonged surgery (i.e. over 3 h) or surgery near the diaphragm.

The stomach produces 1.5 l of gastric secretions (hydrochloric acid, pepsin, water, mucus, etc.) daily, all of which can be lost if an ileus develops. Gastric secretion from the parietal cells in the body and fundus of the stomach is stimulated initially by the vagus nerves through stimuli from the cerebral cortex in response to the thought, smell or taste of food. The hormone gastrin is produced and released by the G-cells of the gastric antrum in response to gastric distension and the presence of the products of digestion. It is transported in the blood stream to the parietal cells which secrete more hydrochloric acid. Large losses of naso-gastric fluid rich in hydrogen ions are a potent cause of metabolic alkalosis.

Normal bowel activity results from a combination of intrinsic and extrinsic innervation as well as chemical stimulation. The bowel has an intrinsic innervation comprising of Meissner's plexus innervating the muscularis mucosae, Aurbach's plexus running between the longitudinal and circular muscle fibres and a serosal plexus between the circular and outer external muscle fibres. Such intrinsic innervation provides the bowel with autonomous muscular activity responsible for mixing and propulsive function.

External innervation is mediated through lumbar splanchnic nerves and responds to mechanical and chemical stimulation. The adrenergic sympathetic component is inhibitory while the parasympathetic component is cholinergic and excitatory. The common causes of intestinal dysfunction are listed in Table 8.1.

Table 8.1 – Causes of gastrointestinal dysfunction following surgery.

Pain and stress
Retro-peritoneal haematoma or intra-peritoneal blood
Infection or inflammation – peritonitis, anastomotic leak, pancreatitis
Metabolic – hypoxia, diabetic ketoacidosis, hepatic encephalopathy, porphyria, hypokalaemia, hypocalcaemia, hypercalcaemia, hypomagnesaemia, hypophosphataemia, acidosis
Immobilisation
Drugs – narcotics, sedatives, anticholinergics, vasoactive agents, psychotropic agents
Endocrine – diabetic gastroparesis, hypothyroidism
Traumatic – surgical manipulation, resection
Mechanical – obstruction at anastomosis, herniation

Not all causes of persistent ileus are easily reversible but they need to be systematically excluded. Large gastric aspirates may occur in the presence of gastric outflow obstruction, or as a result of intestinal ileus or when obstruction causes intestinal fluid to reflux into the stomach. Gastric outflow obstruction is less common than ileus and may be distinguished by the clear colour and high hydrogen ion concentration of the aspirate. Compensatory renal retention of hydrogen ions in exchange for potassium leads to hypokalaemia. Ileus associated with reflux of small bowel contents into the stomach produces a bile stained aspirate. Ileus is associated with loss of water, sodium, potassium and bicarbonate into the small bowel lumen. Duodenal fluid is alkaline with a bicarbonate concentration about twice that of plasma. If bicarbonate loss into the bowel lumen is greater than the rate at which the kidneys can regenerate bicarbonate a metabolic acidosis will develop. Intestinal fluid loss may, therefore, produce vomiting, problems of water loss, electrolyte and acid–base disturbance, ventilatory dysfunction and increased risk of pulmonary aspiration as a result of abdominal distension.

THERAPEUTIC GOALS

The therapeutic goals for this patient are:

1. To improve oxygenation and ventilatory performance.

2. To correct fluid losses and improve cardiovascular function.

3. To correct acid–base disturbance.

4. To encourage mobility.

THERAPEUTIC OPTIONS BASED ON PHYSIOLOGICAL AND PHARMACOLOGICAL EFFECTS

Improve oxygenation and reduce hypoventilation

The patient should be supervised by staff aware of the risks of ventilatory deterioration. Inspired oxygen concentrations of up to 80% can be achieved using a well fitting non-rebreathing mask with a reservoir bag. Loss of sensitivity to carbon dioxide and reliance on hypoxia as the main stimulus to ventilation is suggested by high pre-operative plasma bicarbonate level (i.e. $>30\,mmol.l^{-1}$). In such patients, gradually increasing inspired oxygen concentrations through a fixed performance high flow oxygen entrainment mask should be titrated against observation of the respiratory rate and blood gas analysis (to detect increasing hypercapnia). In our patient, it is vitally important to distinguish between Type II respiratory failure, which is associated with long standing carbon dioxide retention (i.e. COPD), and Type I respiratory failure associated with post-operative atelectasis, sputum retention, abdominal distension, pain, hypokalaemia and hypophosphataemia. Limiting the inspired oxygen concentration may be beneficial in Type II but catastrophic in Type I respiratory failure; Type I (hypoxic) respiratory failure requires correction with inspired concentrations of oxygen high enough to relieve the hypoxaemia.

Other specific measures such as physiotherapy (including incentive spirometry), antibiotics and the patient's usual bronchodilators should be continued. If respiratory function does not improve, early transfer to an intensive care unit for ventilatory support is appropriate. If the patient can co-operate, then a trial of non-invasive ventilation (Chapter 3) together with respiratory stimulants such as doxapram may be sufficient. If this is unsuccessful, then the patient will need tracheal intubation and mechanical ventilation. The pattern of ventilatory support chosen will depend upon whether severe hypoxaemia (Chapter 2) or airflow limitation (Chapter 16) is felt to be the predominant pathophysiological impairment. Epidural analgesia using a combination of an opiate and a local anaesthetic provides better pain relief and less ventilatory depression than parenterally administered opiates and so should be reinstituted.

Gastro-oesophageal reflux and aspiration of gastric contents into the airway is common in critically ill patients. Non-invasive ventilation is associated with gastric inflation and regurgitation of gastric contents and so should be undertaken with caution. Gas swallowing leading to gastric distension is also common. A naso-gastric tube may reduce the volume of gastric contents but may encourage regurgitation by interfering with the gastro-oesophageal sphincter. Microbiological advice should be sought to ensure that appropriate antibiotic treatment is administered.

Fluid and electrolyte imbalance

Normal daily water and electrolyte requirements in an adult are in the region of 2.5 l ($1.5 \, \mathrm{ml.kg^{-1}.h^{-1}}$) together with about 150 mmol ($2 \, \mathrm{mmol.kg^{-1}}$) of sodium and 80–100 mmols ($1–1.5 \, \mathrm{mmol.kg^{-1}}$) of potassium. These requirements will match physiological losses through respiration, in urine and faeces. However, our patient has increased fluid and electrolyte requirements because of surgery, pyrexia and the ileus. Hydration may be assessed by asking about thirst, performing a physical examination and studying the fluid balance charts. The patient's central venous pressure should be interpreted with care as it may not correlate well with intravascular volume and, in this case, may be affected by right ventricular dysfunction secondary to COPD. Dehydration, rather than hypovolaemia, is suggested by levels of serum urea out of proportion to serum creatinine. Osmolality measurement requires a very small volume of plasma or urine and can be done frequently. The normal ratio of urinary to plasma osmolality is greater than $1.1:1$. The ratio will be higher in a dehydrated patient. In acute intrinsic renal failure, any urine produced is isosmolar with plasma because of failure to concentrate the urine. The administration of diuretics, or other drugs that influence urinary sodium excretion will invalidate osmolality estimation and should not be administered until a full assessment of hydration and cardiovascular stability has been completed.

The patient is hypotensive for a man of his age, whose anticipated systolic blood pressure (mmHg) may be estimated as 100 plus his age in years (i.e. about 160 mmHg). He has become oliguric (urine output $<0.5 \, \mathrm{ml.kg^{-1}.h^{-1}}$). Intravascular volume depletion occurs as a result of intra- and post-operative blood loss, pyrexia and sequestration of fluid in tissues and gastrointestinal tract. Intravenous resuscitation with colloid or crystalloid will be required initially to restore circulating volume, cardiac output, arterial blood pressure and renal perfusion pressure. Peri-operative myocardial infarction should be excluded by serial ECGs and enzyme assays. Ileus or mechanical intestinal obstruction may cause symptomatic hypovolaemia and is certain to produce electrolyte and acid–base disturbances. Lactate administered in Hartmann's solution or in haemofiltration replacement fluid may cause elevated lactate levels without an accompanying acidosis. However, persistently elevated lactate levels (i.e. $>2.0 \, \mathrm{mmol.l^{-1}}$) suggest cellular hypoxia. Intravenous fluids should be prescribed with reference to overall fluid balance and

Table 8.2 – Approximate volumes and electrolyte content of gastrointestinal secretions; electrolyte concentrations vary with rate of secretion.

	Volume (ml.day^{-1})	pH	Na$^+$ (mmol.l^{-1})	K$^+$ (mmol.l^{-1})	HCO$_3^-$ (mmol.l^{-1})	H$^+$ (mmol.l^{-1})	Cl$^-$ (mmol.l^{-1})
Saliva	1000	6–7	60	15–30	50	–	15–30
Gastric	1500	1–3.5	50	15	–	150	150
Pancreas	1000	8	140	10	115	–	50
Bile	1000	7–7.4	130	10	10	–	25
Small intestine	1800	7.5–8	140	8	70	–	60–100
Large intestine	200	7.5–8	40	90	30	–	15

values of plasma electrolyte concentrations, 24 h urinary electrolyte excretion and estimations of the electrolyte concentrations in intestinal losses (Table 8.2).

Acid–base balance

At the time of referral, this patient has a mixed acidaemia with a respiratory component caused by the elevated P_aCO_2 at 7.5 kPa and a metabolic component reflected by a base deficit of -12 mmol.l^{-1}. The respiratory component will improve with better alveolar ventilation. The cause of the metabolic component may be related to loss of bicarbonate ions from the small bowel lumen via the nasogastric tube or to the accumulation of non-volatile acids caused by renal dysfunction. Improvement in tissue perfusion, glomerular filtration and effective correction of hypoxaemia usually reverse the metabolic acidosis. However, if this does not occur, renal dysfunction, intra-abdominal sepsis or bowel ischaemia should be suspected.

The interpretation and correction of acid–base abnormalities may be aided by estimating the anion gap. The concept of the anion gap is based on the principle that the sum of the positive and negative charges carried by solutes in body fluids must be equal. Sodium and potassium provide more than 90% of the plasma cation concentration with the balance generated by low concentrations of calcium and magnesium. Over 80% of the plasma anions are chloride and bicarbonate. The remaining 20%, which is usually unmeasured, constitutes the anion gap:

$$\text{Anion gap} = ([Na^+] + [K^+])-([Cl^-] + [HCO_3^-])$$

Because the proportion of unmeasured anions is greater than unmeasured cations, there are more positive charges than negative and the normal anion gap is between 15 and 20 meq.l^{-1} (correct measurement unit is meq because of the polyvalent ions). The anion gap arises because of unmeasured charges on protein and low concentrations of negatively charged urate, sulphate, phosphate and lactate molecules. These represent the non-bicarbonate buffer anions; they are present in the extracellular fluid and glomerular filtrate (except protein) and are important for the excretion of hydrogen ions and the renal regeneration of bicarbonate. An increase in anion gap represents an inability to regenerate bicarbonate ions in the face of a falling plasma bicarbonate concentration. This may occur in lactic or ketoacidosis, in renal failure or in the presence of exogenous molecules such as salicylates, alcohol or ethylene glycol. This additional buffering provided by non-bicarbonate buffers (i.e. proteins, phosphate and sulphate) helps minimise acid–base disturbance until their capacity is exhausted. When this occurs, H^+ concentration increases and pH falls. This patient's anion gap is $17\,\mathrm{meq.l}^{-1}$ suggesting that the main cause of his acidosis is predominantly respiratory.

A refinement of the concept of electrochemical neutrality stems from the suggestion by Stewart that changes in hydrogen ion concentration occur from the variable dissociation of water into $[H^+]$ and $[OH^-]$. This depends on the pK value of water which in turn depends upon the concentrations of ions dissociated in it. Three factors independently influence $[H^+]$: the strong ion difference (SID), the P_aCO_2 and the total weak acid concentration (A_{tot}). A strong ion is one that is almost totally dissociated and the SID is the difference between the sums of the strong cations and anions in solution which may be represented:

$$(Na^+ + K^+ + Ca^{++} + Mg^{++}) - (Cl^- + Lactate^-) = 40 - 42\,\mathrm{mmol.l}^{-1}$$

Note that $[H^+]$ and $[HCO_3^-]$ are weak ions. Weak acids and anionic contributions from albumin and phosphate make up the remaining electrochemical balance. A rise in SID causes less water dissociation and an alkalosis while a fall in SID causes greater dissociation and an acidosis.

Improving intestinal function

A plain abdominal X-ray may assist with the differential diagnosis of ileus and mechanical intestinal obstruction. If an anastomotic breakdown is suspected, the development of a subphrenic abscess, identified by a raised ipsilateral hemi–diaphragm on the affected side, occurs in 80% of patients. Seventy percent of patients with ileus will also show evidence of basal pulmonary consolidation and 60% will have an associated pleural effusion. Expert advice should be sought at the earliest opportunity regarding the interpretation of plain thoracic and abdominal radiographs and the organisation of further appropriate diagnostic imaging such as ultrasound or CT scanning. The evidence to support the use of prokinetic agents such as metoclopramide and erythromycin in post-operative ileus is not compelling.

USUAL OUTCOME

The outcome for this patient depends upon whether his multiple organ failure deteriorates further. On admission to intensive care, he has already developed four-system failure (i.e. cardiovascular, respiratory, gastrointestinal and renal).

This puts his risk of intensive care mortality at approximately 65%. With his pre-existing COPD, weaning from mechanical ventilation via a tracheal tube will be difficult and he will probably require a tracheostomy. If he becomes oliguric and requires renal replacement therapy, then his risk of mortality increases further by 1.5–2 fold. However, provided he develops no further organ failure or complications, his functional status and quality of life should return to pre-operative levels after a prolonged convalescence.

KEY LEARNING POINTS

1. Post-operative deterioration in ventilatory function occurs after abdominal surgery and may cause ventilatory failure in patients with COPD.

2. Hypoxaemia requiring the administration of oxygen develops over the first 48 h post-operatively and persists for up to 10 days.

3. The management of fluid and electrolyte requirements after abdominal surgery should take into account all measurable and insensible losses and requires attention to detail.

4. Urine volume is not necessarily a good guide to renal function.

5. A persistent metabolic acidosis despite treatment may be indicative of an intra-abdominal cause.

6. The primary mechanisms by which disorders of acid–base balance occur should be identified and treated in preference to simple correction of the disturbance itself.

Further reading

1. Dobb GJ, Evans DC, Marshall JC. Disordered gastric motility. In Webb AR, Shapiro MJ, Singer M, Suter P (eds), *Oxford Textbook of Critical Care Medicine.* Oxford: Oxford Medical Publications, 1999: 342–55.

2. Kenny GNC. Risk factors for postoperative nausea and vomiting. *Anaesthesia* 1994; **49**: S6–S10.

3. Mayne PD. Hydrogen ion homeostasis. In Mayne PD (ed.), *Clinical Chemistry in Diagnosis and Treatment – Zilva Pannall Mayne*, 6th edn. London: Arnold, 1994: 80–100.

4. Field S. Plain abdomen. In Armstrong P, Wastie M (eds), *Diagnostic and Interventional Radiology in Surgical Practice.* London: Chapman & Hall Medical, 1997: 15–47.

5. Shelly MP, Nightingale P. Respiratory support. In Singer M, Grant I (eds), *ABC of Intensive Care*. London: BMA publications, 1999: 12–15.

6. Smith AJ, Nissan A, Lanouette NM *et al*. Prokinetic effect of erythromycin after colorectal surgery: randomized, placebo-controlled, double-blind study. *Diseases of the Colon and Rectum* 2000; **43**: 333–7.

7. Story DA, Poustie S, Bellomo R. Quantitative physical chemistry analysis of acid–base disorders in critically ill patients. *Anaesthesia* 2001; **56**: 530–3.

8. Bungard TJ, Kale-Pradhan PB. Prokinetic agents for the treatment of post-operative ileus in adults: a review of the literature. *Pharmacotherapy* 1999; **19**: 416–23.

9

BLEEDING VARICES IN A PATIENT WITH ALCOHOL INDUCED HEPATIC CIRRHOSIS

J Wigfull & A Cohen

CASE SCENARIO

A 45-year-old man, known to Accident and Emergency Department staff, with a history of alcohol abuse, presents following a massive haematemesis. On arrival, he is no longer vomiting and is maintaining his airway. The following observations are made: respiratory rate 30 breaths.min^{-1}, heart rate 105 beats.min^{-1}, arterial blood pressure 80/40 mmHg and Glasgow Coma Scale (GCS) of 9. Initially, he is treated with high flow oxygen via face mask and intravenous fluids via two large peripheral venous cannulae. A secondary survey reveals several spider naevi, a flapping tremor and a palpable spleen. His haemoglobin concentration is 7 g.dl^{-1} and a transfusion of cross-matched packed red cells is started. When stable he is transferred to the endoscopy suite where he becomes agitated and uncooperative. He is given 2 mg intravenous midazolam by the endoscopist. An oesophageal varix is identified as the source of bleeding but 2 min after the midazolam bolus he becomes less responsive with a GCS of 3. He develops airway obstruction and has another large haematemesis.

DEFINITION AND DESCRIPTION OF THE PROBLEM

A patient presenting with massive haematemesis and a depressed level of consciousness will be sensitive to the effects of sedative agents and will require early airway protection and respiratory support. Much of the blood lost may be occult; thus apparent blood loss is an inaccurate guide to volume replacement and aggressive fluid resuscitation will be required. After resuscitation, the patient must be assessed for the presence of encephalopathy, other evidence of impaired liver function and conditions associated with an alcoholic lifestyle such as malnutrition, immuno-suppression and smoking related diseases.

The prevalence of alcoholic cirrhosis is unknown because until the development of liver failure the disease remains clinically silent; however, the incidence is rising in the UK, particularly in the 20–50 age group and in women. Each year, 10% of patients with compensated cirrhosis will decompensate and only 21% of patients survive for 6 years after decompensation. Oesophageal varices are present in 40% of patients at diagnosis of cirrhosis and this increases to 90% after 10 years. Once present, 35% of varices bleed within 2 years; mortality following the first haemorrhage is 50%. The clinical indicators for the risk of variceal bleeding were classified by Child (Table 9.1) but the variceal size and the presence of red spots (sites of recent haemorrhage) on the surface of the varix are also important.

This patient presents with haemorrhage from oesophageal varices and this has caused moderate haemodynamic compromise. He shows signs of chronic liver disease. His reduced conscious level and flapping tremor indicate early encephalopathy making him sensitive to sedatives, including benzodiazepines.

During endoscopy, varices are prone to re-bleeding when manipulated for banding or injection. Ideally, this patient should be endoscoped in theatre under anaesthetic supervision. The decision to protect the airway prior to endoscopy should be made following discussion between senior anaesthetic and gastroenterology staff. This scenario demonstrates poor preparation of a high risk patient, resulting in the need to perform emergency tracheal intubation under difficult conditions. The mortality risk is increased and proper planning could have prevented this situation.

Following neurological deterioration in the endoscopy suite, the patient's trachea was intubated and the bleeding controlled using balloon tamponade; he required transfusion of 16 units of packed red blood cells together with platelets, fresh frozen plasma and cryoglobulin.

Table 9.1 – Child's classification of risk of bleeding within 1 year. These are mean values. Actual risk varies according to size of the varices and the presence of red spots on the surface of the varix.

	Child's class		
	A	B	C
Risk of bleeding (%)	10	30	65
Serum bilirubin (mg.l^{-1})	<20	20–30	>30
Serum albumin (g.l^{-1})	>35	30–35	<30
Ascites	None	Easily controlled	Poorly controlled
Neurological disorders	None	Minimal	Severe
Nutrition	Excellent	Good	Poor

PATHOLOGY AND PATHOPHYSIOLOGY OF PROBLEM

Alcoholic liver disease

Alcohol is directly hepatotoxic and induces both fibrogenesis (secondary to inflammation) and necrosis of hepatocytes. Ethanol and its metabolites can also directly activate fibrogenesis and affect collagen metabolism. Cirrhosis is defined by the World Health Organisation as 'a diffuse process characterised by fibrosis and the conversion of the normal liver architecture into structurally abnormal nodules.' This process occurs because the relationship between hepatocytes and the extracellular matrix, which contains collagen, is disturbed. Hepatocyte necrosis is followed by regeneration which necessitates new matrix formation. When regeneration is significant, lobular architecture is disturbed resulting in nodules. The formation of intrahepatic shunts reduces vascularity and so increases resistance to portal blood flow. At a microscopic level, the composition of the new matrix favours the formation of dense bundles of collagen. The distribution of matrix deposition is altered and peri-sinusoidal fibrosis occurs in the space of Disse. In the chronically damaged liver, matrix production is stimulated whilst degradation is inhibited so that the process may become self-perpetuating.

As resistance to portal flow increases, portal hypertension develops. The portal pressure gradient can be estimated by measuring the hepatic venous pressure gradient – the difference between wedged and free hepatic venous pressure (normal values are 3–6 mmHg). Collateral circulation develops through channels that open as a result of the increased hydrostatic pressure; a threshold hepatic venous pressure gradient of 10 mmHg is thought to be necessary. It is not known whether angiogenesis also contributes to collateral formation. Clinically, the most significant collaterals are those that drain to the azygos and hemiazygos veins via gastro-oesophageal varices.

Portal-systemic encephalopathy

Portal-systemic (hepatic) encephalopathy is a complex neuropsychiatric syndrome, the mechanisms of which are still poorly understood. Major disturbances occur in the GABA-ergic (gamma-aminobutyric acid), glutamatergic and glutaminergic systems. Hyperammonaemia associated with liver failure is central to these disturbances. Synergistic toxins (e.g. mercaptans, phenols, short-chain fatty acids) potentiate the effects of ammonia in the brain. False neuro-transmitters may be formed because increased aromatic amino acids and decreased branched-chain amino acids favours the entrance of the former into the brain. Ammonia, however, is not a specific indicator of encephalopathy and it can be normal in significant hepatic coma; the level does not correlate well with the degree of coma, but levels $>200 \text{ mg.l}^{-1}$ increase the risk of cerebral oedema formation.

Raised concentrations of ammonia result in multiple effects on both inhibitory and excitatory pathways, but over time there is a degree of compensation. This explains

Table 9.2 – Clinical grading system for hepatic encephalopathy.

Grade 1
Mild confusion, euphoria, depression, poor attention, slurred speech, irritability, reversed sleep pattern, slowed mental tasks

Grade 2
Lethargy, inappropriate behaviour, drowsy, obvious personality changes, intermittent disorientation, incontinence, worse at mental tasks

Grade 3
Somnolent but rousable, unable to perform mental tasks, disorientated and confused, amnesia, fits of rage, incoherent speech

Grade 4
Coma with response to pain (4a), without response to pain (4b)

why the clinical signs are often a mixture of central nervous system depression and excitation and why chronic encephalopathy differs from that seen in fulminant hepatic failure. Increases in intracranial pressure (ICP) caused by astrocyte swelling may occur. The clinical grading of encephalopathy is given in Table 9.2 while the factors that can precipitate encephalopathy are shown in Table 9.3.

Table 9.3 – Factors precipitating acute hepatic encephalopathy in cirrhotic patients.

Most common
- Gastointestinal haemorrhage
- Uraemia
- Sedative drugs
- Diuretics

Other causes
- Dietary protein load
- Infection
- Constipation
- Electrolyte imbalance, especially hypokalaemia

If no precipitating factor is found
- Deterioration in liver function
- Increasing porto-systemic collateral circulation

Several effects of hyperammonaemia occur:

1. Ammonia directly stimulates $GABA_A$ receptors to cause neuronal depression. It also has a direct effect on astrocytes causing swelling and an increase in the number of peripheral benzodiazepine receptors. These effects result in increased production of neurosteroids which are potent endogenous agonists of $GABA_A$ receptors. The synaptic GABA concentration increases due to down regulation of $GABA_B$ receptors and reduced re-uptake by astrocytes.

2. The glutamatergic system is stimulated by calcium dependant glutamate release which results from nerve depolarisation, a direct consequence of hyperammonaemia. NMDA (N-methyl-D-aspartate) stimulation is exacerbated by inhibition of the endogenous NMDA antagonist kynurenic acid. Excessive NMDA stimulation causes excitotoxicity and irreversible neuronal injury.

3. Glutamine is synthesised in astrocytes from ammonia and glutamate catalysed by glutamine synthetase. Astrocyte swelling is largely prevented by inhibition of this enzyme suggesting glutamine contributes to the raised ICP. Glutamine/tryptophan counter exchange across the blood brain barrier promotes neural serotonin synthesis which may reach a toxic concentration. Drugs affecting monoamine synthesis and re-uptake, such as antidepressants, should be stopped.

Massive transfusion

Whole blood is no longer available in the UK for clinical use. In the following discussion 'blood' refers to red blood cells re-suspended in saline, adenine, glucose and mannitol (SAGM) solution. In countries where whole citrated blood is still used it must be remembered that citrate toxicity is more likely in liver disease and that activity of platelets and some clotting factors (especially Factors V and VIII) diminish rapidly. A transfusion is conventionally considered 'massive' when the patient's normal circulating blood volume is replaced within 24 h.

Complications of a massive transfusion include:

1. Idiopathic and incompatibility reactions and pathogen transmission. These complications are not directly associated with volume, but have an accumulative risk associated with each unit transfused.

2. Complications associated with blood storage are also important.

    •   Blood is refrigerated and should be administered via a blood warmer, particularly if the patient has other risk factors for hypothermia (e.g. prolonged surgery or collapse). Moderate hypothermia promotes a diuresis via inhibition of tubular re-absorption and anti-diuretic hormone release. Severe hypothermia may promote a coagulopathy.

    •   Microaggregate formation during storage is reduced, but not eliminated, by mannitol. Transfusion of microaggregates results in pulmonary microemboli that may account for the hypoxaemia sometimes seen after large volume blood transfusions. Blood should be administered via a 'blood giving set' which has a mesh filter size of approximately 170 μm, although this will only remove larger aggregates. Smaller aggregations can be removed using a 40 μm filter but such fine filters may induce further cell damage. The evidence does not support the use of 40 μm filters.

- During storage, red cells continue to metabolise substrate, which is energy dependant (hence the presence of adenine and glucose in SAGM). After three weeks storage, the pH is lower, and ammonia levels up to nine times higher, than normal; fresh blood should preferentially be given to patients at risk of hepatic encephalopathy if available. As substrate is depleted, potassium leaks out of the cells and membrane integrity cannot be maintained resulting in stiff, brittle cells. The intracellular concentration of 2,3-diphospho-glycerate (2,3-DPG) is reduced. Storage dependent changes result in several deleterious processes. The acid and potassium load may result in cardiovascular compromise. The temperature, acid load and 2,3-DPG depletion cause a leftward shift in the oxygen dissociation curve. The poor rheological properties result in reduced capillary flow and further cell damage.

3. Dilutional effects.

- Platelets and clotting factors are lost along with red cells during haemorrhage, then consumed in an attempt to effect haemostasis before being diluted by resuscitation with clear fluids. This patient's clotting times and platelet count may already be abnormal as a result of liver disease and he is at risk of disseminated intravascular coagulation. During active bleeding the platelet count should be kept above $50 \times 10^9 \, l^{-1}$. Fresh frozen plasma is given if the International Normalised Ratio (INR) is raised and cryoglobulin is given if fibrinogen is depleted (e.g. $<1.0 \, g.l^{-1}$). There is no evidence to support the use of prophylactic clotting factors when indices of coagulation are normal. Dilution of white cells during transfusion does not occur to a significant extent because of their naturally short-life span and the extensive bone marrow reserves. Transfusion of white blood cells is not indicated during active, fluid resuscitation; indeed, blood in the UK is now depleted of white cells in an attempt to reduce risk of prion transmission.

4. Other adverse effects of massive transfusion include fluid overload and respiratory impairment, but these are covered in Chapters 1 and 2 respectively. For the reasons detailed above, patients who receive large volumes of stored blood require frequent assessment of serum electrolytes, arterial blood gases, full blood count and clotting. The frequency of sampling will depend on the rate of transfusion.

THERAPEUTIC GOALS

The therapeutic goals in this patient include:

1. Resuscitation using ABC guidelines with particular attention to volume replacement.

2. Identification of the source of bleeding. There are a number of therapeutic options to stop bleeding or to reduce the risk of a re-bleed.

3. Minimise risk of decompensation by limiting the risk of developing ascites and hepatic encephalopathy.

THERAPEUTIC OPTIONS BASED ON PHYSIOLOGICAL AND PHARMACODYNAMIC EFFECTS

Resuscitation

Massive variceal bleeding must be treated aggressively according to current Airway–Breathing–Circulation protocols. Transfusion requirements are often large and the need for platelets, fresh frozen plasma and cryoglobulin common. Massive transfusion is liable to cause electrolyte abnormalities, particularly hyperkalaemia and hypocalcaemia. The aims of resuscitation after variceal bleeding are: restoration of systolic arterial pressure to 90–100 mmHg, restoration of haematocrit to 25–30% and the maintenance of an adequate urine output ($0.5 \, ml.kg^{-1}.h^{-1}$). The central venous pressure should be monitored to guide fluid resuscitation. If fluid resuscitation is excessive the portal pressure will rise increasing the risk of re-bleeding.

Endoscopy

Endoscopy is indicated as soon as the patient has been adequately resuscitated, so that useful diagnostic and prognostic information can be provided prior to balloon tamponade or surgery. Rapidly bleeding varices make endoscopy technically difficult. Occasionally, blood loss is so brisk that, to prevent exsanguination, control by balloon tamponade cannot be delayed. Sclerotherapy involves injecting a sclerosant into or adjacent to the varix. This causes thrombus formation in or inflammation around the vessel; both result in reduced variceal flow. Variceal band ligation is as effective in controlling acute haemorrhage and has fewer side-effects. Injection of acrylate glue is a new endoscopic option, but its place in emergency haemorrhage control is not established.

Pharmacological therapy

Splanchnic vasoconstrictors such as vasopressin, somatostatin, and their analogues, have been used to reduce portal flow. Vasopressin is a potent vasoconstrictor which has a high incidence of side-effects related to systemic vasoconstriction (e.g. myocardial ischaemia, arrhythmias and cerebrovascular accidents). Terlipressin is a synthetic analogue of vasopressin that has a longer half-life, provides improved control of bleeding and causes fewer side-effects. Somatostatin, and its analogue octeotride, also effectively control bleeding. Somatostatin is as effective as terlipressin in the control of bleeding (approximately 80%) and has fewer side-effects; however, to date, terlipressin is the only drug proven to reduce mortality. Octeotride theoretically causes less splanchnic vasoconstrition than vasopressin and despite paucity of published evidence it is extensively used.

Other drugs used in patents suffering a gastrointestinal haemorrhage include antibiotics, lactulose and anti-emetics. Prophylactic antibiotics should be given for 7 days to all cirrhotic patients presenting with haematemesis to reduce the risk of spontaneous bacterial peritonitis and bacteraemia. Quinolones are commonly used for selective decontamination of the digestive tract (SDD); oral norfloxacin (400 mg twice daily) has been the most extensively studied and its efficacy repeatedly demonstrated. Lactulose is given to keep the bowel empty, reducing absorption of highly nitrogenous compounds such as blood. Many patients require anti-emetic therapy. Metoclopramide and domperidone increase the lower oesophageal sphincter tone and have the theoretical advantage of reducing flow in the azygos vein. However, neither drug has been shown to control bleeding or reduce re-bleeding when used alone.

Sodium retention, due to activation of the renin–angiotensin system, contributes to expansion of the circulating blood volume and, consequently, increases portal pressure; ascites will also be exacerbated. Once bleeding has been controlled, the sodium content of feed and intravenous fluids should be kept to a minimum. Single diuretics, combinations of loop diuretics and spironolactone, or diuretics and angiotensin converting enzyme inhibitors have all been used to promote a negative sodium balance.

Balloon tamponade

Balloon tamponade is used to achieve temporary haemostasis, whilst alternative strategies are commenced. Its efficacy is highly variable (e.g. 40–90% temporary control) and should only be used for 24 h to avoid mucosal ulceration. Approximately 50% of patients re-bleed within 24 h after balloon deflation. Several types of tubes with different arrangements of balloons are available. In the UK, the four lumen Sengstaken Blakemore tube, which has oesophageal and gastric balloons and aspiration channels is commonly used; current practice is to inflate the gastric balloon for both gastric and oesophageal varices as compression at the gastro-oesophageal junction lowers the intravascular pressure at the bleeding site allowing clot formation. Inflation of the oesophageal balloon is associated with a higher complication rate. Protocols vary but typically the gastric balloon is inflated with 300 ml of air and the tube position checked radiologically before external traction is applied, using a 0.5 kg weight for 50 min in each hour.

Surgery and interventional radiology

Several forms of shunt surgery have been used in the past and have largely been replaced by the formation of a transjugular intrahepatic porto-systemic shunt (TIPS), which effectively diverts blood away from the liver but increases the risk of developing encephalopathy. The TIPS procedure is used for patients who re-bleed following endoscopic and pharmacological therapy. On the basis of current evidence, it is not recommended for prevention of variceal haemorrhage. Cirrhotic patients may ultimately require transplantation (Table 9.4).

Table 9.4 – Indications and contraindications for liver transplantation.

Indications for liver transplantation
Disease state
   Advanced chronic liver disease
   Acute liver failure
   Hepatocellular carcinoma without extrahepatic spread
   Others (rare)
Immediate requirement for transplantation (e.g. fulminant hepatic failure)
Estimated 1-year survival <90%
Child class B or C
Portal hypertensive bleeding or spontaneous bacterial peritonitis (regardless of Child's class)
No alternative treatment
Appropriate psychological profile to comply with long-term care
Consent

Contraindications to liver transplantation
Extrahepatic malignancy
Sepsis
Severe cardiopulmonary disease
Alcohol or drug abuse within 6 months
Compensated cirrhosis without complications (Child's class C)
Technically impossible to transplant (e.g. anatomical abnormality)

Prevention of re-bleeding

A combination of beta blockade and variceal ligation are used once the acute bleed has resolved.

USUAL OUTCOME

The majority of patients with variceal haemorrhage are managed on medical wards or high-dependency units. Patients are often referred to the intensive care unit for airway protection to avoid the risk of aspiration resulting from reduced conscious level. A patient should be considered at risk if the GCS is 8 or less. Pneumonitis secondary to aspiration of blood is commonly seen. Those admitted to intensive care represent a subpopulation with severe disease in whom outcome is poor. Most acute hospitals are able to resuscitate patients and provide appropriate endoscopic and pharmacological treatment. Transplantation is not appropriate during the acute setting and the most likely reason to transfer patients to a regional centre is for a TIPS.

KEY LEARNING POINTS

1. Airway compromise is the most common reason for referral to intensive care.

2. Rapid infusion of large volumes of intravenous fluid and blood are required, but excessive resuscitation increases the risk of re-bleeding.

3. Prophylactic measures should be initiated to reduce the risks of re-bleeding. The most effective regimen is constantly changing with the results of new research.

4. Decompensation and encephalopathy may be limited or prevented by gut decontamination, judicious use of blood products and nutrition. Further haemorrhage remains the greatest risk factor.

Further reading

1. Guadalupe G. Current management of the complications of cirrhosis and portal hypertension: variceal hemorrhage, ascites, and spontaneous bacterial peritonitis. *Gastroenterology* 2001; **120**: 726–48.

2. Albrecht J, Jones EA. Hepatic encephalopathy: molecular mechanisms underlying the clinical syndrome. *Journal of Neurological Sciences* 1999; **170**: 138–46.

3. Bircher J, Benhamou J-P, McIntyre N, Rizzetto M, Rodes J. *Oxford Textbook of Clinical Hepatology*, 2nd edn. Oxford: Oxford University Press, 1999.

4. Keeffe E. Liver transplantation: current status and novel approaches to liver replacement. *Gastroenterology* 2001; **120**: 749–62.

5. Soderlund C, Magnusson I, Torngren S, Lundell L. Terlipressin (triglycyl-lysine vasopressin) controls acute bleeding oesophageal varices. A double-blind, randomized, placebo-controlled trial. *Scandinavian Journal of Gastroenterology* 1990; **25**: 622–30.

10

DROWNING AND CEREBRAL HYPOXIA

D Sim & W Woodward

CASE SCENARIO

A 20-year-old man is brought to the Accident and Emergency (A&E) Department having been rescued from the bottom of a public swimming pool. Basic life support was performed by lifeguards, but a paramedic ambulance crew arriving within 10 min found the victim pulseless and apnoeic; the defibrillator monitor showed ventricular fibrillation. Sinus rhythm was restored after three DC shocks, but the patient remained unresponsive and was intubated at the scene without sedation or paralysis. He was manually ventilated, and upon arrival in A&E, he was still unresponsive and had fixed dilated pupils. Breath sounds were heard bilaterally and although he felt cold, a weak carotid pulse was palpable (heart rate: 55 beats.min^{-1}). As he was moved onto the A&E trolley, his pulse became impalpable, and pulseless electrical activity (PEA) was diagnosed. Cardiac massage was commenced, and after 3 min and 1 mg of intravenous adrenaline, spontaneous circulation returned transiently before reverting to PEA again.

DEFINITION AND DESCRIPTION OF THE PROBLEM

Near-drowning is defined as an episode of asphyxiation in fluid that results in a period of survival following the incident. In the UK in 1998, near-drowning accounted for almost 400 hospital episodes. Drowning may occur in the home or garden, in swimming pools or in open water. Other injuries (e.g. cervical spine fractures) may also occur and immobilisation of the neck in a hard collar following rescue is vital. Near-drowning is often associated with alcohol or the use or overdose of prescription and non-prescription drugs. A primary neurological or cardiac event (e.g. seizure, myocardial infarction or primary arrhythmia) may also be the initiating cause. Rarely, drowning may be secondary to attempted suicide. A full history should be sought from any available witnesses.

The primary determinant of outcome following near-drowning is the occurrence of circulatory arrest. Survival in individuals who maintain spontaneous circulation is greater than 98%, but falls to 20% in those requiring cardiopulmonary resuscitation (CPR). In the latter group, outcome depends on early application of effective life support and so is improved by bystander CPR. Hypothermia is a common feature of near-drowning in non-tropical waters, particularly in thermally unprotected individuals. However, hypothemia has both beneficial and adverse effects. There is little doubt that profound hypothermia confers neurological protection during circulatory arrest. There are many reports of cerebrally intact survivors of prolonged submersion. In particular, small children, who cool more quickly, and those rescued from colder waters, may have unexpectedly good outcomes. However, restoration of spontaneous circulation may not be possible until core temperature has been restored to at least 30°C (see below), and CPR should continue until either the victim is warmed to 35°C or until rewarming is judged to be unachievable.

Indicators of poor outcome include dilated unreactive pupils and asystole on arrival at hospital, and a Glasgow Coma Scale (GCS) score below 6 on admission to intensive care. Unfortunately, all early signs are unreliable in predicting death or severe disability. However, if neurological function remains poor with no sign of improvement 24 h after restoration of a stable circulation, death or severe impairment are the most probable outcomes.

PATHOLOGY AND PATHOPHYSIOLOGY OF THE PROBLEM

When submersion in water occurs, initial voluntary breath holding may be accompanied by the diving reflex. This is seen more often in young children and babies and consists of bradycardia, apnoea and intense peripheral vasoconstriction resulting in preferential blood flow to the heart and brain. At the breakpoint of breath holding, involuntary gasping occurs and water inhalation leads to laryngeal spasm. Vomiting may occur, and then a period of secondary apnoea is followed by further gasps, which may result in aspiration of water. Unconsciousness and death is inevitable without rescue. If the victim is rescued from the water and resuscitated, widespread physiological disturbance can be expected.

Central nervous system

Primary hypoxic brain injury occurs at the time of the original insult, and irreversible cell death will begin within 5 min of inadequate cerebral oxygen delivery. Secondary brain injury can arise at any stage after the primary insult and is due to decreased oxygen delivery to injured and oedematous areas of brain. Significant primary brain injury will result in cerebral oedema, peaking in severity between 24 and 72 h after the initial event. Brain swelling, severe enough to increase intracranial pressure (ICP), will reduce cerebral perfusion pressure (cerebral perfusion pressure = mean arterial pressure − ICP) and thereby exacerbate secondary brain injury.

Cardiovascular system

Cardiac arrest occurs secondary to hypoxaemia, or occasionally as a primary event causing the near-drowning. Any arrhythmia may be seen after near-drowning, particularly, in the presence of hypothermia. The ECG in hypothermia characteristically shows bradycardia with PR and QT interval prolongation, progressing to complete heart block at lower temperatures. Below 28°C, refractory ventricular fibrillation commonly supervenes; this is often precipitated by physical stimuli such as turning. A characteristic positive deflection after the QRS complex (the J-wave) appears below 33°C (Figure 10.1).

Above 33°C, shivering artefact may complicate ECG interpretation. Following successful resuscitation, ECG and cardiac enzyme testing may reveal signs of myocardial injury. Low cardiac output with intense, global vasoconstriction

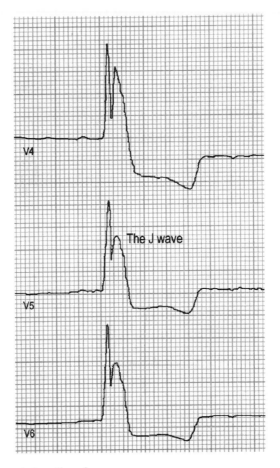

Figure 10.1 – J-waves in hypothermia.

following resuscitation is exacerbated by hypothermia and severe acidaemia. The systemic inflammatory response syndrome (SIRS) may occur later due to the hypoxic insult or secondary to injury to other organs, particularly the lungs. A cascade of inflammatory mediators released by neutrophils and endothelial cells leads to abnormal circulatory regulation at a local level with low systemic vascular resistance, impaired perfusion and organ dysfunction.

Respiratory system

Aspiration of water, whether salt or fresh, leads to both immediate and delayed lung injury. Although post-mortem examinations of drowned victims often show only a limited amount of water in the lungs, it is likely that water is rapidly absorbed across the alveolar membrane. Immediate local effects of aspiration include bronchospasm, abnormal blood flow distribution and pulmonary oedema. Ventilation–perfusion mismatch and arterial hypoxaemia develop.

Although there may be theoretical differences in the initial effects of fresh and salt water on the lungs with regard to fluid absorption, both fluids lead to surfactant damage with reduced compliance and areas of alveolar collapse. Damage to the alveolar capillary membrane leads to increased capillary permeability with non-cardiogenic pulmonary oedema. This may progress to acute lung injury or the acute respiratory distress syndrome (ARDS). Vomiting and aspiration of gastric contents may also occur. In patients requiring positive-pressure ventilation, high-inflation pressures are often needed due to bronchospasm and low-pulmonary compliance, so risking barotrauma (Chapter 2).

Infection, occasionally with unusual pathogens, may develop after aspiration of contaminated water, or secondary to ventilator associated pneumonia. Evidence for the benefit of prophylactic antibiotics and steroids in pulmonary aspiration is lacking.

Renal system

Hypothermia reduces renal tubular sodium reabsorption and decreases collecting duct sensitivity to anti-diuretic hormone (ADH). These effects combine to produce an increased output of dilute urine despite reduced cardiac output and glomerular filtration rate. This 'cold diuresis' may contribute to hypovolaemic shock. Hypoxic damage sustained during and after immersion may lead to acute anuric renal failure, despite subsequent restoration of renal oxygen supply.

Gastrointestinal system

Hypoxaemia leads to liver and bowel injury, which may not initially be clinically evident. Transaminase enzyme rises suggest hepatocellular damage, while an increasing prothrombin time points to progressive liver dysfunction. Bowel necrosis presents with bloody diarrhoea, and refractory metabolic acidosis often with hyperlactataemia.

Haematologic changes

Freshwater aspiration may cause haemolysis of red cells as the hypotonic fluid is absorbed into the circulation. This rarely causes a clinical problem, although significant haemoglobinaemia may precipitate renal failure. Both hypothermia and hypoxic injury cause bone marrow suppression with low white cell and platelet counts. Coagulation times are prolonged by hypothermia, and intravascular coagulopathy occurs in response to endothelial dysfunction associated with the inflammatory response.

THERAPEUTIC GOALS

The aims of immediate therapy following near-drowning are:

1. Initiate support of airway, breathing and circulation.

2. Commence rewarming using peripheral and core techniques as appropriate.

3. Prevent secondary brain injury by providing optimal conditions for cerebral oxygen delivery.

4. Supportive treatment for acute lung injury and other organ system failures.

THERAPEUTIC OPTIONS BASED ON PHYSIOLOGICAL AND PHARMACODYNAMIC EFFECTS

Airway

In an unconscious near-drowning victim, airway management includes tracheal intubation both for airway protection and mechanical ventilation; the position of the tracheal tube is confirmed clinically initially and later radiologically. Muscle rigidity in profound hypothermia is unresponsive to neuromuscular blockade and by limiting mouth-opening may make orotracheal intubation impossible. The risks of vomiting or regurgitation of gastric contents and subsequent aspiration are high. Foreign matter should be cleared from the airway, but the Heimlich manoeuvre (i.e. an abdominal thrust) is not indicated, unless the airway cannot be cleared adequately from above. Cervical spine immobilisation is vital, where an injury is possible. High concentration inspired oxygen should be administered.

Breathing

While respiratory support may be provided initially with manual self-inflating resuscitation bag, mechanical ventilation is usually required. Bronchospasm causes increased airway resistance with high inflation pressures; bronchodilators can be nebulised into the ventilator circuit, but may be ineffective. Peripheral pulse oximetry probes usually give inaccurate readings due to poor peripheral circulation. Adequacy of oxygenation and ventilation and the degree of metabolic acidosis are assessed by arterial blood gas analysis. However, hypothermia complicates interpretation. Actual oxygen and carbon dioxide tensions are lower than in a sample analysed at 37°C owing to their increased solubility. The pH is higher and the normal range of values at 37°C do not apply since cellular metabolic function is depressed at low temperatures. Buffering processes and oxyhaemoglobin dissociation are also substantially altered. Despite these factors, it is generally accepted that interventions based on P_aCO_2 and pH *corrected to 37°C* are appropriate. However, it must be appreciated that actual P_aO_2 at the patient's temperature is less than that measured at normothermia, so as to avoid missing significant hypoxaemia.

Hypoxaemia is usually due to a combination of ventilation–perfusion mismatch and pulmonary oedema. Ventilation to a P_aCO_2, approximately 4.5 kPa, is appropriate in order to maintain normal cerebral blood flow without increasing ICP. Once mechanical ventilation is established, addition of positive end-expiratory pressure (PEEP) is likely to be necessary to achieve adequate oxygenation. The potential benefits of high levels of PEEP (i.e. >15 cmH$_2$O) in improving oxygenation must be balanced against deleterious effects on venous return, with reduced cardiac output and increased ICP. In severe refractory hypoxaemia, ICP monitoring along with pulmonary artery catheterisation or flow-directed circulatory management may be needed to optimise the ventilatory pattern.

Chest X-ray may show bilateral alveolar infiltrates consistent with pulmonary oedema, due to left-ventricular failure, ARDS, or a combination of both. In ARDS, inverse ratio ventilation and prone positioning improve oxygenation, although neither have improved mortality. Inhaled nitric oxide, nebulised prostacyclin, high frequency oscillation and haemofiltration are also unproven therapies when oxygenation becomes critical.

Circulation

Management of the circulation is difficult in hypothermic immersion victims. Even central pulses may be difficult to feel and where doubt exists, external cardiac massage should be continued. The chest wall may be rigid and effective compressions difficult. ECG monitoring is essential, and dysrhythmias should be treated along current advanced life support guidelines. However, it is important to be aware of the confounding effects of hypothermia on drug actions and electrical treatment such as pacing and defibrillation. Establishing intravenous access may be difficult or impossible and the intraosseous route should be considered early, even in adults.

In the presence of severe metabolic acidosis (i.e. pH < 7.0), intravenous sodium bicarbonate is often given at a dose of 1 mmol.kg^{-1} (i.e. 1 ml.kg^{-1} of 8.4%

bicarbonate solution). Although alkalising agents have not been shown to improve survival, myocardial performance is impaired by severe acidosis.

Once spontaneous circulation returns, invasive arterial monitoring is a priority. Central venous access should also be obtained as soon as possible. The first circulatory intervention is volume replacement, but inotropic drugs (e.g. dobutamine) should be started if cardiac output remains inadequate. During the initial resuscitation, adrenaline solution $100\,\mu g.ml^{-1}$ $(1:10\,000)$ can be administered into a large vein starting at $2-5\,ml.h^{-1}$ for an adult.

Impaired ventricular function may be secondary to ischaemic myocardial injury combined with the effects of hypothermia and acidaemia. Vasodilatation during rewarming causes hypotension, but it may also herald the onset of the SIRS. Failure of the circulation to respond predictably to fluid loading, an escalating inotrope requirement, or widening base deficit are indications for more detailed circulatory assessment. Echocardiography, pulmonary artery catheterisation and oesophageal Doppler all provide useful information about intravascular volume status, cardiac output and vascular tone, and guide fluid and inotrope therapy. However, arrhythmias may be precipitated by any invasive monitoring technique.

Rewarming

Restoration of body temperature is a key aspect of management of the hypothermic immersion victim. A 60 kg subject with an average specific heat capacity of $0.83\,kcal.kg^{-1}.°C^{-1}$ requires 300 kcal of heat energy to raise the body temperature from 28°C to 34°C. Techniques chosen depend on the severity of hypothermia and the presence or absence of spontaneous circulation (Table 10.1).

There are two important issues:

1. In circulatory arrest below 28°C, the myocardium must be raised to a defibrillatable temperature as quickly as possible. This can only be achieved through active core (central) warming, and most efficiently using extracorporeal circulation.

2. Following return of spontaneous cardiac output, a uniform return of body temperature towards normothermia is desirable. However, avoiding the problems of excessive vasodilatation with rapid flux of inflammatory mediators from hypoperfused areas, hypotension, acidosis and secondary re-cooling is a challenge. Less invasive active external warming may be employed at this stage. Shivering thermogenesis, occurring between 30°C and 35°C, increases heat production dramatically, but at a severe oxygen cost and with the risk of anaerobic metabolism and hyperlactataemia.

Passive external warming is the least invasive approach and relies on methods of insulating the patient. Metabolic thermogenesis produces a gradual temperature

Table 10.1 – Rewarming techniques.

Technique	Comments
Passive	
Remove wet clothing, dry skin, shelter from wind and insulate with blankets	Average rate of temperature rise $<0.5°C.h^{-1}$; useful for mild hypothermia or pre-hospital situation
Active	
Peripheral (external)	
Forced air warming blanket, warm water bath and hot water bottles	Difficult to control; incidence of serious complications may be higher when periphery warmed before core in profound hypothermia ($<28°C$)
Central (core)	*Ascending order of invasiveness*
Warmed humidified inspired gases ('cascade' humidifier)	Maximum 45°C: delivers $10\,kcal.h^{-1}$; effective and safe
Warmed intravenous fluids	Maximum 40°C: delivers $10\,kcal.l^{-1}$ (all routes)
Warmed gastrooesophageal lavage; bladder irrigation; pleural cavity lavage via chest drains	All intracavitary methods may precipitate venticular fibrillation
Warmed peritoneal lavage or dialysis	Potassium-free dialysate, 40°C, short-dwell time
Extracorporeal circulation	Haemofiltration circuit delivers $\cong 120\,kcal.h^{-1}$ at $200\,ml.min^{-1}$; cardiopulmonary bypass obviates need for CPR and affords the most effective control over rewarming rate (up to $3000\,kcal.h^{-1}$) and metabolic fluxes, for example, potassium

rise, but is only suitable for mild to moderate hypothermia (i.e. $>32°C$) in conscious individuals.

Metabolic

Severe metabolic acidosis is common after near-drowning and is usually accompanied by high-serum lactate levels due to a combination of cardiac arrest or low cardiac output and hypothermia. Lactic acidosis will normally correct spontaneously over several hours following restoration of tissue oxygen delivery. Persistent metabolic acidosis despite adequate volume replacement and cardiac function suggests renal or liver impairment or ischaemic bowel.

Various electrolyte abnormalities are seen in near-drowning episodes. Following freshwater immersion, absorption of hypotonic fluid into the circulation may cause hyponatraemia, which is usually self-limiting. Severe hyperkalaemia (serum potassium over $10\,mmol.l^{-1}$) may develop rapidly following rewarming, reperfusion and rhabdomyolysis. Renal replacement therapy (e.g. haemofiltration) may be necessary to control potassium if life threatening arrhythmias supervene.

Hyperglycaemia is common during the initial resuscitation stage, but should not be treated if the victim is hypothermic; blood glucose usually returns to normal, once the patient is rewarmed and stabilised. Persistent hyperglycaemia ($>10\,mmol.l^{-1}$) should be controlled to prevent worsening of secondary brain injury to a level of $5–10\,mmol.l^{-1}$ using an intravenous insulin sliding scale.

Renal

A urinary catheter should be inserted during the resuscitation phase. The polyuria of cold diuresis may cause or unmask hypovolaemia and must be treated aggressively. Acute renal failure developing subsequently will require continuous renal-replacement therapy, if the patient becomes anuric.

Gastrointestinal tract

A nasogastric tube should be inserted during the resuscitation phase. Once stabilised on the ICU, enteral nutrition should be started early unless ischaemic bowel is suspected (e.g. worsening metabolic acidosis, increasing lactate and bloody diarrhoea). Resection of non-viable bowel is not appropriate, if ischaemia is widespread. Hypoxic liver injury usually improves spontaneously after restoration of oxygen delivery.

Infection

Pulmonary infection may develop following aspiration of infected material, or due to ventilator associated pneumonia. Pyrexia, leucocytosis and raised C-reactive protein levels indicate, but do not confirm, invasive infection. A systemic inflammatory response following the initial insult may produce a similar clinical picture in the absence of infection. Conversely, severe sepsis may further impair an immune response already depressed as a result of the initial insult, and the above clinical features may not be obvious. Positive microbiological cultures from blood, sputum and other sites are treated along conventional lines. Prophylactic antibiotics, generally, are not used as they are likely to lead to selection of resistant organisms. The use of corticosteroids in pulmonary aspiration is controversial.

Central nervous system

Initial assessment of the central nervous system includes pupil size and reactivity, GCS and blood glucose level. The effects of hypothermia and depressant drugs should be taken into account and a blood alcohol level measured and urine sent for toxicology. The neurological state of the patient during the initial phase of resuscitation may indicate, but does not reliably predict, outcome. If adequate circulation is re-established and the patient remains unresponsive, support on intensive care should be continued for at least a further 24 h to allow more reliable and detailed assessment of central nervous system function. Death or severe disability is more probable if, at 24 h, purposeful movements are absent or there is evidence of abnormal brain stem function. A CT scan of the brain is necessary to exclude a primary intracranial event and look for features of hypoxic brain injury (e.g. loss of grey–white matter differentiation).

Seizure activity must be controlled promptly, initially with benzodiazepines and phenytoin loading. In refractory or subclinical convulsive states, barbiturate infusions may be required, but their long duration of action delays full neurological assessment. Myoclonus is a poor prognostic sign.

Cerebral oedema following hypoxic brain injury may increase ICP, so impairing cerebral perfusion. While ICP monitoring has not been shown to improve outcome after drowning, the information it provides may be valuable in guiding therapy. The use of short acting sedative drugs by infusion, and neuromuscular blockade if ICP is critical, reduce cerebral oxygen demand without delaying neurological assessment unduly. Maintaining mild hypothermia (33–35°C) may afford some cerebral protection, but the resulting cardiovascular instability and shivering will negate any benefits, if not prevented. The established principles of nursing the patient in a 30° head-up position, maintaining the mean arterial pressure at the patient's normal level, and P_aCO_2 around 4.5 kPa, should be followed. Venous congestion from tracheal tube tie, head position, or cervical collar should be avoided.

BRAIN STEM DEATH

A relentless rise in ICP consequent upon primary and secondary brain injury ultimately forces the cerebellar tonsils into the foramen magnum at the skull base (i.e. coning). This results in compression of the brain stem and later irreversible cessation of its function; brain stem death has been considered synonymous with the death of the individual since 1976. Where brain stem death has been diagnosed using rationally agreed guidelines, no individual has ever recovered and cardiac standstill usually occurs within a few days. In patients diagnosed as brain stem dead, organ donation may be considered. Appropriate patients include those with fatal brain injury secondary to trauma, haemorrhage or circulatory arrest. There is no upper age limit for organ donation.

Diagnosis of brain stem death

Testing is performed by two doctors, at least one of whom must be a consultant, and the other registered for at least 5 years. They should be competent in their field and not members of a transplant team. Four preconditions must be met before brain stem death testing can be carried out. These, and the tests performed, are shown in Table 10.2.

The oculovestibular reflex text may be omitted, if prevented by severe head trauma. The absence of respiratory effort can be demonstrated by delivering oxygen via a suction catheter passed down the tracheal tube to maintain oxygenation during apnoea, while watching for movement of the chest and diaphragm. P_aCO_2 normally increases at approximately $0.3\,kPa.min^{-1}$ during apnoea, but may climb more slowly in brain stem dead individuals in whom metabolism is slowing. The P_aCO_2 must be confirmed by measurement of arterial blood gases. The persistent spinal reflexes following brain stem death may be distressing for relatives and staff, and should be carefully explained.

Table 10.2 – Diagnosis of brain stem death.

Preconditions
The patient must be unconscious with a known irreversible cause of coma.
No residual drug effects contributing to CNS depression or paralysis.
No endocrine or metabolic disturbance causing CNS depression.
No primary hypothermia – core temperature >35°C.

Tests (numerals indicate cranial nerves tested)
Absence of pupillary light reflexes (II, III).
Absence of corneal reflexes (V).
Absence of oculovestibular reflexes (VIII, III) – no eye movement following injection of 50 ml icy water into the external auditory meatus (normal response – nystagmus with fast component away from the ear tested). The tympanic membranes must first be inspected to confirm external auditory canal patency.
Absence of motor responses within the cranial nerve distribution to any central or peripheral stimuli (V, VII).
Absence of gag and cough reflexes (e.g. carinal stimulation with a suction catheter (IX, X)).
Absence of respiratory efforts despite an arterial P_aCO_2 exceeding 6.65 kPa (50 mmHg) when disconnected from the ventilator for at least 5 min.

Two sets of tests are carried out and may be performed by the two doctors together or separately. There is no fixed time interval between the two sets of tests. The legal time of death is when the first set of tests is completed, but death is pronounced following the second set.

Suitability for organ donation

Although donated organs must be functioning and free from disease, a period of hypoxaemia or cardiac arrest does not necessarily render the organs unsuitable for transplant. General exclusions include transmissible systemic infection, malignancy other than primary brain tumours, type 1 diabetes mellitus, autoimmune disease, a history of intravenous drug abuse or risk factors for human immunodeficiency virus (HIV) infection. Heart valves, corneas, bone and skin can be donated up to 24 h after asystole, but other organs must have the minimum possible ischaemic time (i.e. time between removal from the donor and transplant into recipient).

Consent for organ donation

Consent for organ donation is sought from next of kin. This difficult issue must be approached in a sensitive but timely manner. Not infrequently, the subject of organ donation is raised by the relatives themselves. If known, the patient's pre-morbid wishes should be taken into account. Sensitive enquiry about the donor's lifestyle is necessary, including agreement to HIV testing.

Involvement of Her Majesty's Coroner

Where death was not due to natural causes, and particularly following trauma or assault, the agreement of the coroner is necessary for organ harvest to proceed. However, the nature of the injuries rarely prevents donation. The coroner's appointed pathologist may be present at the time of surgery and a post-mortem may be performed after organ removal is completed.

Procedure

Once brain stem death has been confirmed and relatives have agreed for organ donation, the local transplant coordinator should be informed. The coordinator is responsible for ensuring suitability of the donor, tissue typing, location of potential recipients via the national register and liaising with the transplant teams. Any doubt regarding suitability of organs can be resolved through discussion with transplant teams, possibly with further investigations.

A comprehensive array of investigations includes a full range of biochemical and microbiological tests, HIV, hepatitis and other viral serology and tissue typing. These procedures normally take several hours and the time interval between identification of a donor and harvesting organs is usually in the order of 12–24 h, as retrieval teams may need to travel some distance from the tertiary transplant centres.

Management of the organ donor

Maintenance of oxygenation and optimal organ perfusion are the main aims underlying management of the organ donor. Thus, ventilation and circulatory support should continue as before brain stem death, but additional problems are likely to develop.

Cardiovascular system

Cardiovascular instability may occur due to the central effects of brain stem death. Hypotension occurs in around 80% of brain stem dead patients, and aggressive fluid loading may be necessary. The loss of central sympathetic output leads to peripheral vasodilatation. Inotropes are avoided if possible, especially if the heart is to be donated; but can be used if needed to maintain organ perfusion. The transplant team may recommend particular inotropes according to their own protocols. Arrhythmias are treated along standard lines, but management should not normally extend to CPR unless organ harvest is imminent. If haemodynamic deterioration leads to circulatory arrest, the retrieval teams must be notified immediately.

Respiratory system

P_aO_2 should be maintained at or greater than 10 kPa using the lowest possible inspired oxygen concentration. Neurogenic pulmonary oedema may compromise oxygenation and modest levels of PEEP (5–10 cmH$_2$O) are acceptable.

Endocrine and metabolic changes

Hypothermia is common following brain stem death and is due to loss of central hypothalamic control compounded by peripheral vasodilatation and heat loss. It will contribute to cardiovascular instability and arrhythmias, if not treated. Forced air warming is normally sufficient to maintain body temperature and more active methods may be required (Table 10.1).

Cranial diabetes insipidus is a frequent feature of brain stem death. Loss of ADH leads to a high output of dilute urine and resultant hypernatraemia. DDAVP, a synthetic analogue of ADH, in a dose of 2 μg intravenously or subcutaneously, effectively controls the excessive diuresis.

Cortisol production decreases due to loss of pituitary output of adreno-corticotrophic hormone (ACTH). This can contribute to hypotension, necessitating replacement with intravenous hydrocortisone. Thyroid function may also be depressed, and administration of tri-iodothyronine is occasionally requested by the transplant teams. Blood glucose should be maintained at normal levels using an insulin infusion, if necessary.

Haematological

Disseminated intravascular coagulation occurs in 25% of brain stem dead patients and is due to release of cerebral thromboplastins after brain death. Fresh frozen plasma may be needed, particularly during organ harvesting.

USUAL OUTCOME

Outcome from drowning is difficult to predict on the basis of neurological function at presentation to hospital, but is generally worse in those with prolonged immersion, prolonged CPR, asystole at presentation and absent spontaneous movement or abnormal brain stem reflexes at 24 h.

Resuscitation should continue until rewarming is achieved, and organ support maintained until formal neurological assessment after at least 24 h. Treatment is supportive and no specific additional interventions have been shown to alter outcome. Those diagnosed brain stem dead should be considered for potential organ donation. Organ donation procedures are well established and should be followed.

KEY LEARNING POINTS

1. The primary determinant of outcome from near-drowning is the occurrence of circulatory arrest.

2. Hypothermia is a common feature of near-drowning in non-tropical waters, particularly, in thermally unprotected individuals.

3. Restoration of spontaneous circulation may not be possible until core temperature has been restored to at least 30°C, and CPR should continue until the victim is warmed to 35°C or rewarming is judged to be unachievable.

4. Indicators of poor outcome include dilated unreactive pupils and asystole on arrival at hospital, and a GCS below 6 on admission to intensive care.

---

5. Primary hypoxic brain injury, cardiac arrest secondary to hypoxaemia and acute lung injury are the predominant clinical problems.

6. Initial management of near-drowning focuses on the restoration of oxygen delivery.

7. The possibility of cervical spine and other trauma must be considered.

8. If adequate circulation is re-established and the patient remains unresponsive, support on intensive care should be continued for at least a further 24 h to allow more reliable and detailed assessment of central nervous system function. Death or severe disability are more probable if, at 24 h, purposeful movements are absent or there is evidence of abnormal brain stem function.

9. Victims diagnosed brain stem dead should be considered for potential organ donation. Organ donation procedures are well established and should be followed.

Further reading

1. Department of Health. *Hospital Episode Statistics.* London: Department of Health, 1998.

2. Simcock AD. Drowning and near drowning. In Driscoll P, Skinner D (eds), *Trauma Care: Beyond the Resuscitation Room.* London: BMJ Publishing, 1998, 249–54.

3. Bossaert L, Van Hoeyweghen R. Bystander cardiopulmonary resuscitation (CPR) in out-of-hospital cardiac arrest. *Resuscitation* 1989; **17**: S55–S69.

4. Lopez-Pison J, Pineda-Ortiz I, Oteiza C *et al.* Survival with no sequelae after near-drowning with very poor signs for prognosis including persistent bilateral non-reactive mydriasis. *Revista de Neurologia* 1999; **28**: 388–90.

5. Siebke H, Rod T, Breivik H, Link B. Survival after 40 minutes submersion without cerebral sequelae. *Lancet* 1975; **1** (7919): 1275–7.

6. Lavelle JM, Shaw KN. Near drowning: is emergency department cardiopulmonary resuscitation or intensive care unit cerebral resuscitation indicated? *Critical Care Medicine* 1993; **21**: 368–73.

7. Spack L, Gedeit R, Splaingard M, Havens PL. Failure of aggressive therapy to alter outcome in pediatric near-drowning. *Pediatric Emergency Care* 1997; **13**: 98–102.

8. Miyake M, Iga K, Izumi C, Miyagawa A, Kobashi Y, Konishi T. Rapidly progressive pneumonia due to *Aeromonas hydrophila* shortly after near-drowning. *Internal Medicine* 2000; **39**: 1128–30.

9. Wilichowski E, Christen HJ, Schiffmann H, Schulz-Schaeffer W, Behrens-Baumann W. Fatal Pseudallescheria boydii panencephalitis in a child after near-drowning. *The Pediatric Infectious Disease Journal* 1996; **15**: 365–70.

10. Chugh KS, Sitprija V, Jha V. Tropical Countries. In Davison AM, Cameron JS, Grunfeld J-P (eds), *Oxford Textbook of Clinical Nephrology*. Oxford: Oxford University Press, 1998: 1726.

11. Walpoth BH, Locher T, Leupi F *et al.* Accidental deep hypothermia with cardiopulmonary arrest: extracorporeal blood rewarming in 11 patients. *European Journal of Cardiothoracic Surgery* 1990; **4**: 390–3.

12. Myers RA, Britten JS, Cowley RA. Hypothermia: quantitative aspects of therapy. *Journal of the American College of Emergency Physicians* 1979; **8**: 523–7.

13. Bratton SL, Jardine DS, Morray JP. Serial neurologic examinations after near drowning and outcome. *Archives of Pediatric and Adolescent Medicine* 1994; **148**: 167–70.

14. Torbey MT, Selim M, Knorr J, Bigelow C, Recht L. Quantitative analysis of the loss of distinction between gray and white matter in comatose patients after cardiac arrest. *Stroke* 2000; **31**: 2163–7.

15. Hachimi-Idrissi S, Corne L, Huyghens L. The effect of mild hypothermia and induced hypertension on long term survival rate and neurological outcome after asphyxial cardiac arrest in rats. *Resuscitation* 2001; **49**: 73–82.

16. Hicks SD, DeFranco DB, Callaway CW. Hypothermia during reperfusion after asphyxial cardiac arrest improves functional recovery and selectively alters stress-induced protein expression. *Journal of Cerebral Blood Flow and Metabolism* 2000; **20**: 520–30.

17. Working Group of Conference of the Medical Royal Colleges and their Faculties in the United Kingdom. Diagnosis of brain death. *Lancet* 1976; **ii**: 1069–70.

18. Intensive Care Society. *Donation of Organs for Transplantation. The Management of the Potential Organ Donor*. London: Intensive Care Society, 1999.

11

SEVERE HAEMORRHAGE AFTER CAESARIAN SECTION IN A PRIMIGRAVIDA

R Meacher & S Brett

CASE SCENARIO

A previously fit 24-year-old primigravida, with recently diagnosed pre-eclampsia, is admitted to the intensive care unit (ICU) following Caesarian section. Surgery was performed at 36 weeks gestation because of rising blood pressure, worsening headaches, visual disturbances and epigastric pain. It was performed under general anaesthesia, as the platelet count was low at $60 \times 10^9 l^{-1}$ and regional blockade was contraindicated. Other than methyldopa for hypertension, the patient takes no medication and has no known allergies.

Following delivery, severe haemorrhage developed and eventually the uterus was packed. Blood loss was estimated as 6 l and she was transfused 10 units of packed red cells, 2 units of fresh frozen plasma (FFP) and one pooled donation of platelets. A radial arterial line and an internal jugular central line have been inserted.

On admission to the ICU, she is pale and cold, with a pulse of 120 beats.min^{-1} and a blood pressure of 110/76 mmHg. Blood is slowly oozing from the line sites and into the surgical drains. She remains intubated and ventilated. She is oliguric.

DEFINITION AND DESCRIPTION OF THE PROBLEM

Typically, blood loss at Caesarian delivery is between 900 and 1100 ml, although clinical estimates of blood loss are unreliable. When defined as a 10% drop in haematocrit or the need for transfusion, obstetric haemorrhage complicates 6.4% of Caesarian section deliveries. With severe haemorrhage, intra-operative resuscitation of the mother continues while surgical attempts are made to arrest the bleeding. However, after massive transfusion, coagulopathy occurs and worsens any underlying bleeding tendency. Surgical efforts are made more difficult and a vicious cycle of bleeding and coagulopathy ensues. In the ICU, fluid resuscitation and correction of the coagulopathy are essential. Continuing haemorrhage may require further surgery.

As in this case, obstetric haemorrhage is often associated with an underlying disorder. Pre-eclampsia is defined as the combination of hypertension (diastolic pressure >110 mmHg on one occasion or >90 mmHg on two occasions) with proteinuria (>300 mg in 24 h) in a pregnant woman of more than 20 weeks gestation. It is a multi-system disorder affecting 5.8% of primigravidas and 0.4% of second pregnancies. The classic presentation is with hypertension, proteinuria and oedema, although many other features may be present (Table 11.1).

Eclampsia is a life threatening complication and may progress from pre-eclampsia, although in 38% of women, seizures are the presenting feature. Forty-four per cent of seizures occur in the post-partum period. Other causes of obstetric haemorrhage should be considered. Amniotic fluid embolism, placental abruption and sepsis typically cause disseminated intra-vascular coagulation (DIC). Amniotic fluid embolism causes acute respiratory failure and rapid circulatory collapse; it has a mortality of over 60%. Treatment is supportive. Haemorrhagic problems may also be caused by inherited disorders of coagulation, the most common being von Willebrand disease, in which there is a quantitative or qualitative abnormality of

Table 11.1 – Clinical features of pre-eclampsia.

Hypertension
Diastolic >110 mmHg
Systolic >160 mmHg*
Proteinuria
Oedema and excessive weight gain
Hyperuricaemia
Hypoalbuminaemia
Oliguria and acute renal failure*
Pulmonary oedema*
Epigastric or right upper quadrant pain*
Abnormal liver function tests*
Hepatic rupture*
Cerebral signs: headache, blurred vision or altered consciousness*
Eclampsia*
Thrombocytopaenia
HELLP syndrome*

*Features of severe eclampsia.

von Willebrand factor, which normally promotes platelet adhesion to damaged endothelium.

The normal physiological changes in pregnancy result in an increase in coagulation factors, a reduction in fibrinolysis and hence an increased risk of thrombosis. The risk of thrombosis is even higher following operative delivery and, therefore, prophylaxis against deep vein thrombosis must be started as soon as the coagulopathy has resolved and haemostasis is achieved.

PATHOLOGY AND PATHOPHYSIOLOGY

Haemorrhage at Caesarian section occurs predominantly from the uterus. The spiral arteries of the placenta are denuded of their muscular layer as part of the physiological adaptation to pregnancy, and occlusion of these vessels after delivery depends on uterine contraction. The risk of haemorrhage from the placental bed is increased by uterine atony caused by amnionitis, prematurity, arrested labour, general anaesthesia with volatile agents and, possibly, magnesium infusions. Pre-eclampsia doubles the risk of haemorrhage. Structural abnormalities such as placenta previa, placenta accreta and placental abruption are also significant causes of haemorrhage.

Massive transfusion can be defined as the replacement of the whole blood volume within 24 h or more than 50% of the blood volume within 1 h. The side effects of massive transfusion are given in Table 11.2. With coagulopathy, brisk small vessel bleeding is seen in the operative field and oozing occurs from puncture sites. Dilutional coagulopathy develops because stored red cells are deficient in functional platelets and coagulation factors; thus, transfusion dilutes the patient's remaining coagulation reserves. These dilutional effects are exacerbated by the infusion of fluids other than blood or blood products. Hypothermia resulting from the rapid transfusion of cold blood also worsens coagulation. Dilutional coagulopathy associated with massive transfusion occurs when blood loss and its replacement exceeds one blood volume. The platelet count typically falls below $50 \times 10^9 l^{-1}$ only when

Table 11.2 – Side effects of massive transfusion.

Metabolic changes
    Alkalosis: due to citrate toxicity (used as an anticoagulant and converted to bicarbonate)
    Acidosis: stored blood has a pH of 6.9 due to preservatives
    Hyperkalaemia: potassium leakage from red cells results in potassium concentration in
      stored blood of up to 20 mmol.l^{-1}
    Hypocalcaemia: calcium chelated by citrate
    Leftward shift of O_2 dissociation curve: caused by low 2,3-diphosphoglycerate levels in
      transfused red blood cells
Acute lung injury or acute respiratory distress syndrome: infusion of micro-aggregates
Hypothermia
Coagulopathy: dilutional

Table 11.3 – Changes in test results associated with haemostatic defects.

Defect	Platelet count	PT	APTT	TT	Fibrinogen level	D-dimers
Dilutional defect	↓	↑↑	↑↑	→	↓	Absent
DIC	↓↓	↑↑	↑↑	↑↑	↓↓	Present

PT, prothrombin time; APTT, activated partial thromboplastin time; TT, thrombin time; D-dimers, fibrinogen-degradation products.

more than 1.5 blood volumes are lost. Mobilisation of platelets from the lungs and spleen may help to preserve the circulating platelet pool in the first instance. Laboratory results that differ from a dilutional pattern (Table 11.3) may suggest additional pathologies.

The aetiology of pre-eclampsia is unknown but is associated with placental abnormalities and the release of factors that damage maternal vascular endothelial cells. The damaged endothelium produces pro-coagulants and vasoconstrictors resulting in platelet aggregation and vasospasm. Increased responsiveness to circulating vasoconstrictors, such as angiotensin II, worsens vasospasm and further reduces organ perfusion. Capillary permeability is increased, causing peripheral oedema, and may be a causative factor in the development of pulmonary oedema.

In addition to hypertension and labile blood pressure, the usual cardiovascular changes in pre-eclampsia are a reduction in plasma volume, low central venous pressure (CVP) and low or normal pulmonary capillary wedge pressures (PCWP). Left ventricular contractility is usually unchanged with a raised systemic vascular resistance. In severe pre-eclampsia, there is often little correlation between CVP and PCWP. After delivery, mobilisation of extra-vascular fluid to the intra-vascular compartment may result in fluid overload and pulmonary oedema. However, pulmonary oedema is more commonly due to excessive intravenous fluid administration or the acute respiratory distress syndrome as part of multi-organ failure.

Oliguria and a raised serum creatinine, are common findings and are secondary to reduced renal perfusion and glomerular filtration. Swelling of the glomeruli and fibrin deposition on endothelial cells (glomerular capillary endotheliosis) are present and occasionally progress to acute renal failure. Hepatic dysfunction can occur in pre-eclampsia due to hepatic necrosis, subcapsular haemorrhages or fibrin deposition. Liver rupture is a rare but life threatening event.

Cerebral oedema, haemorrhages and micro-infarcts have been demonstrated on CT imaging of the brain in eclamptic women. Neurological symptoms such as headache, visual disturbances, hyper-reflexia and fitting may be secondary to these effects. Cerebral vasospasm probably plays a role in the development of the ischaemic changes and may explain why magnesium, a potent vasodilator, is effective at controlling seizures.

Mild thrombocytopaenia is common in pregnancy and pre-eclamptic women and has little effect on bleeding. Severe thrombocytopaenia (platelet counts below $100 \times 10^9 1^{-1}$) affects 15% of those with pre-eclampsia and is associated with abnormal tests of coagulation in 7%. This thrombocytopaenia may be due to a low grade DIC with widespread activation of coagulation, intra-vascular formation of fibrin, and consumption of coagulation factors and platelets. Thrombotic occlusion of small and midsize vessels may contribute to multi-organ failure. Fibrinolysis is increased in the later stages of DIC. The diagnosis of DIC is based on laboratory findings (Table 11.3) including thrombocytopaenia, marked hypofibrinogenaemia and the presence of D-dimers.

It is now thought that many cases of thrombocytopaenia in pre-eclampsia are a form of micro-angiopathic haemolytic anaemia (MAHA). This differs from DIC in that the primary defect is endothelial damage with resulting adhesion and aggregation of platelets, thrombin formation, and secondary activation of the clotting cascade. Haemolysis occurs as red cells are distorted as they pass through thrombosed blood vessels. Deficiency of a specific protease that affects von Willebrand factor has been demonstrated.

The syndrome of *h*aemolysis, *e*levated *l*iver enzymes and *l*ow *p*latelets (HELLP syndrome) complicates 4% of cases of severe pre-eclampsia and can present with abdominal pain, nausea, vomiting and jaundice. The haemolysis (a form of MAHA) can be diagnosed by the presence of fragmented red blood cells in the blood film, anaemia and increased serum haptoglobins or lactic dehydrogenase. Coagulation disturbances occur in 20% of cases and nearly 8% progress to acute renal failure.

Amniotic fluid embolism usually occurs at delivery, when amniotic fluid enters the maternal circulation, probably via the placental margin. Amniotic fluid contains foetal debris, cellular material and lipids that have a thromboplastin-like activity on the coagulation cascade. A severe haemorrhagic disorder develops with uncontrolled bleeding. Occlusion of the pulmonary micro-circulation with emboli may result in acute respiratory distress and cardiovascular collapse.

THERAPEUTIC GOALS

The therapeutic goals in this patient are aimed to:

1. Continue resuscitation with fluids and blood products to normalise haemodynamics and improve organ perfusion. This can be guided by clinical signs and invasive monitoring.

2. Aggressively correct the coagulopathy with blood products and treatment of any underlying cause. Close liaison with the Haematology Department and frequent assessment of the coagulation profile is required.

3. Monitor the patient closely for continued bleeding that may necessitate further surgical intervention, especially, if the coagulopathy has been corrected.

4. Minimise the risk of complications such as sepsis and thrombosis. Further complications of pre-eclampsia such as fitting, acute respiratory distress syndrome and renal failure may occur post-partum.

THERAPEUTIC OPTIONS BASED ON PHYSIOLOGICAL AND PHARMACOLOGICAL EFFECTS

Resuscitation

Fluid resuscitation should continue in order to replace the existing deficit and any continuing losses, and to provide maintenance fluid requirements. Blood pressure is particularly a poor guide to volume status in young patients as compensatory mechanisms maintain blood pressure in the presence of severe hypovolaemia. Although normotensive, this patient has a tachycardia and signs of vasoconstriction; these signs are consistent with a reduction in plasma volume of at least 1 l. Furthermore, in the absence of adequate fluid resuscitation, hypovolaemia will become even more apparent on re-warming. There is no convincing evidence to determine the type of fluid used in resuscitation. Colloids remain in the circulation for longer than crystalloids, but gelatins may cause anaphylaxis and interfere with the administration of blood products. High molecular weight hydroxyethyl starches can impede clotting. The repeated administration of saline infusions can result in a hyperchloraemic metabolic acidosis, which has also been implicated in clotting dysfunction. Frequent estimations of haemoglobin can guide blood transfusion, although the choice of target haemoglobin is arbitrary; many ICUs use a target haemoglobin concentration of $8 \, \text{g.dl}^{-1}$ in young previously fit patients.

The amount of intravenous fluid required can be judged using clinical signs and invasive monitoring. Pulse, blood pressure, peripheral perfusion and capillary refill time should be regularly assessed. Urine output should be maintained at greater than $0.5 \, \text{ml.kg}^{-1}.\text{h}^{-1}$. A low CVP confirms hypovolaemia, but a normal or high value does not exclude the need for further fluid. It is often necessary to assess the CVP response to a fluid challenge ($\sim 200 \, \text{ml}$ bolus) when other signs suggest hypovolaemia. The use of a pulmonary artery catheter and measurement of PCWP can give a better guide to filling status, but insertion is more risky in the presence of coagulopathy. The oesophageal Doppler probe is less invasive and can be used to assess cardiac output and filling. Raised base deficit and serum lactate levels suggest anaerobic metabolism and inadequate organ perfusion.

In pre-eclampsia, fluid resuscitation is complicated by the pre-existing low blood volume and the lack of correlation between CVP and PCWP. Oliguria may be present despite resuscitation and urine output may not reflect the adequacy of the circulatory volume. Treating oliguria with repeated fluid challenges is unwise, unless ventricular filling pressures are monitored. However, in the setting of massive haemorrhage, hypovolaemia is more likely and more dangerous than fluid overload. Relative hypertension may be required to maintain cerebral perfusion in the presence of cerebral oedema especially as cerebral autoregulation is lost.

Correction of coagulopathy

The transfusion of blood products, such as FFP and platelet concentrates, should ideally be guided by laboratory results, although empirical treatment is sometimes required. Tests of coagulation must be repeated at regular intervals until the coagulopathy is corrected and haemostasis is achieved. Close liaison with haematology staff is advised. FFP, a source of coagulation factors, can be infused at 1 unit per 10 kg body weight, if the prothrombin and activated partial thromboplastin times are prolonged. Cryoprecipitate is rich in fibrinogen and is used when fibrinogen levels are disproportionately low ($<1.5\,g.l^{-1}$). Platelet concentrates should be given to maintain a platelet count of greater than $50 \times 10^9\,l^{-1}$. One unit of platelets per 10 kg body weight is infused. Each unit of platelets should increase platelet counts by $10 \times 10^9\,l^{-1}.m^{-1}$ of body surface area. Whole fresh blood contains both plasma and platelets but is no longer readily available. Six units of platelets contain approximately 300 ml of plasma. The prophylactic use of platelets and plasma during transfusion has not been shown to reduce transfusion requirements. However, during continuing massive transfusion, requirements for blood products must be anticipated. It is logical to administer platelet and clotting factors simultaneously, so that all necessary components of coagulation are present together. Most obstetric units now have 'massive obstetric haemorrhage' packs agreed with their haematology colleagues and available for rapid release.

The treatment of DIC is usually supportive, although in some cases treatment of the underlying condition will reverse DIC. Low dose heparin infusion at a rate of $500\,u.h^{-1}$ has been advocated by some groups, particularly, in the management of DIC associated with placental abruption and amniotic fluid embolus. Anti-fibrinolytic agents (e.g. aprotinin and tranexamic acid) may worsen intra-vascular thrombosis and result in clot formation in unwanted sites. The role of recombinant anti-thrombin III remains unclear.

Specific treatment of uterine bleeding

Medical management

Prostaglandins and oxytocics can be used to induce uterine contraction and minimise blood loss from the placental bed. Oxytocin, a naturally occurring polypeptide from the posterior pituitary, binds to specific receptors on myometrial cells. Synthetic oxytocin (syntocinon) is given as an initial intravenous bolus of 10 units followed by infusion at a rate to control haemorrhage. Forty units can be added to

500 ml of normal saline. Side effects include vasodilation, reflex tachycardia and coronary ischaemia. The half-life of syntocinon is short at 1–7 min. In large doses, it has an antidiuretic effect, and has been associated with pulmonary oedema. Ergometrine, an ergot alkaloid with powerful oxytocic effects, can be given in combination with syntocinon. However, it can induce severe nausea and vomiting. Its use is contraindicated in pre-eclampsia due to its sympathomimetic effects.

Carboprost (15-methyl prostaglandin F2*a*) is a prostaglandin analogue used to treat uterine atony in patients unresponsive to oxytocics. In primary post-partum haemorrhage, it stops bleeding in 90% of patients. However, its use at Caesarian section is not proven to be superior to syntocinon. It is given in 250 µg boluses by repeated deep intramuscular injection, at intervals of 15–90 min to a maximum dose of 2 mg. Side effects include fever, bronchospasm and hypertension and, therefore, it must be used with caution in pre-eclampsia. Injection directly into myometrium has been advocated, but is of no proven benefit.

Surgical management

In the presence of normal coagulation, continued bleeding warrants further surgical intervention. Uterine packing with gauze may be effective, but it must be removed after 24–36 h at which time bleeding may recur. The use of an intra-uterine balloon (the gastric balloon of a Sengstaken–Blakemore tube or Foley catheter) can be used to compress the myometrium in a similar fashion. Bilateral ligation of the internal iliac arteries controls haemorrhage in only 50% of cases, as pelvic collaterals continue to supply the uterus. Stepwise uterine devascularisation involves progressive ligation of vessels. A new technique of angiographic embolisation of internal iliac, uterine, ovarian or pudendal arteries requires considerable radiological expertise. All these techniques avoid hysterectomy, and thus retain fertility, but surgical complications can occur and unless the relevant expertise is immediately available, hysterectomy may be safer and quicker.

Prevention of complications

Continuing transfusion of cold blood causes hypothermia and is prevented by fluid warmers. Prophylactic antibiotics can reduce the incidence of sepsis as a result of packs left *in situ*. Current recommendations advise the use of anti-thromboembolism stockings in combination with low dose heparin in women undergoing Caesarian section. This should be commenced when initial resuscitation is completed. Other complications such as renal failure are best prevented by adequate resuscitation.

In pre-eclampsia, recurrent hypertension can be controlled with agents such as labetalol (a combined α- and β-adrenergic receptor blocker) given by infusion at 20–160 mg.h^{-1}. Oral α- or β-adrenergic receptor blockers may also be useful. The vasodilator hydralazine can be infused at 5–20 mg.h^{-1} following an initial 5 mg bolus. Nitrate vasodilators are used less frequently, although in the post-partum period there are no concerns about foetal toxicity.

The prophylactic use of anti-convulsants remains controversial. Their use is often reserved for patients with symptoms such as headache and hyper-reflexia suggestive of cerebral involvement and impending seizures. Magnesium sulphate is the agent of choice, both for prophylaxis and treatment. It is given by infusion to achieve a therapeutic concentration of $2-3.5\,mmol.l^{-1}$. Plasma levels greater than $4\,mmol.l^{-1}$ are associated with toxicity. Frequent monitoring of plasma concentrations and assessment of tendon reflexes for hyporeflexia should be performed.

The use of corticosteroids in the post-partum period results in a more rapid increase in the platelet count, urine output and resolution of haemolysis in the HELLP syndrome. Dexamethasone 5 mg twice daily reduces the requirement for platelet transfusions.

USUAL OUTCOME

Major obstetric haemorrhage is now unusual in the developed world and with correct management, rarely results in death. However, pre-eclampsia contributes to 10% of maternal deaths in the UK, and the HELLP syndrome carries a 1–4% mortality. The recurrent risk of pre-eclampsia and the HELLP syndrome have been reported as approximately 40% and 20%, respectively. Women should be counselled about future pregnancies.

KEY LEARNING POINTS

1. Life threatening massive haemorrhage can occur at Caesarian section and requires prompt resuscitation and continued management on the ICU.

2. Dilutional coagulopathy following massive transfusion can be complicated by other causes of abnormal bleeding such as DIC. The pattern of changes in coagulation tests can indicate aetiology. Whatever the cause, treatment is with supportive component therapy.

3. Further pharmacological and surgical therapy may be required to bring bleeding under control.

4. Treatment of any underlying disorder is mainly supportive, only in a few cases specific therapy is required to prevent complications.

5. The outcome of severe haemorrhage is usually good. Mortality is more often related to underlying conditions such as pre-eclampsia.

Further reading

1. Drife J. Management of primary postpartum haemorrhage. *British Journal of Obstetrics and Gynaecology* 1997; **104**: 275–7.

2. Mushambi MC, Halligan AW, Williamson K. Recent developments in the pathophysiology and management of pre-eclampsia. *British Journal of Anaesthesia* 1996; **76**: 133–48.

3. Martlew VJ. Perioperative management of patients with coagulation disorders. *British Journal of Anaesthesia* 2000; **85**: 446–55.

4. Reiss RF. Hemostatic defects in massive transfusion: rapid diagnosis and management. *American Journal of Critical Care* 2000; **9**: 158–65.

5. Levi M, de Jonge E, van der Poll T, ten Cate H. Novel approaches to the management of disseminated intravascular coagulation. *Critical Care Medicine* 2000; **28**: S20–S24.

12

SEVERE ABDOMINAL PAIN DUE TO ACUTE-ON-CHRONIC PANCREATITIS

J Kinsella & T Quasim

CASE SCENARIO

A 44-year-old man is admitted to the surgical ward with severe abdominal pain and vomiting. The pain, has lasted several days, is central, radiates to the back and is similar to, but more severe than, that experienced during several previous episodes. He has a history of cigarette smoking and heavy alcohol consumption, and has been on a 2-day drinking bout the previous weekend. He has a history of ischaemic heart disease and takes occasional nitrates and Fluvastatin 40 mg daily for hypercholesterolaemia.

His temperature is 38.2°C. He has a tachycardia (120 beats.min^{-1}), is hypotensive (90/55 mmHg) and tachypnoeic (22 breaths.min^{-1}). He has a distended abdomen with mild abdominal tenderness and guarding. Peri-umbilical and flank discolouration are also noted and a provisional diagnosis of acute pancreatitis is made. In the next 24 h, he is given 6 l of intravenous fluids and 60% oxygen via a face mask. However, his arterial blood pressure remains low (95/50 mmHg) and he remains hypoxaemic ($P_aO_2 = 8$ kPa) despite oxygen therapy. Consequently, he is referred to the intensive care unit (ICU).

DEFINITION AND DESCRIPTION OF THE PROBLEM

Acute pancreatitis may be difficult to diagnose as it shares many clinical features with other upper abdominal pathology. Differential diagnoses include peptic ulceration, cholecystitis, bowel ischaemia and obstruction. Pancreatitis may also be confused with extra-abdominal causes of pain, including myocardial ischaemia.

The diagnosis of pancreatitis is based on the following:

History

A characteristic symptom is persistent upper abdominal pain, radiating in a band to the back, associated with vomiting. Abdominal distention and tenderness in the epigastric region is usual. Less commonly, more widespread tenderness or pain in the left or right upper quadrant may be present.

Examination

Patients may be generally unwell, but if the pancreatitis is severe, can present with multiple-organ dysfunction or failure. Clinical signs suggestive of pancreatitis include a distended abdomen with epigastric discomfort and both peri-umbilical (Cullen's sign) and flank (Gray Turner's sign) discolouration. Such discolouration indicates extensive retroperitoneal fat necrosis and haemorrhage, a feature of severe pancreatitis. In addition, the Systemic Inflammatory Response Syndrome (SIRS) may develop. A diagnosis of SIRS is based on at least two of the following criteria: a temperature above 38°C or below 36°C; a white blood count above 12 or below $4 \times 10^9 l^{-1}$; a heart rate above 90 beats.min^{-1} or tachypnoea above 20 breaths.min^{-1} or a low P_aCO_2.

Biochemical markers and scoring systems

Serum levels of pancreatic enzymes, such as amylase or lipase, are frequently used to support the presumed diagnosis. However, amylase is non-specific, being found in organs such as the salivary glands or fallopian tubes, and its serum level increases in other abdominal emergencies (e.g. perforated viscus or peritonitis). Amylase is excreted by kidney and, therefore, its level may be raised in renal failure. In addition, the increase in serum amylase level depends on the aetiology of the pancreatitis, with a smaller rise in hypertriglyceridaemia-associated disease. Also, despite being high during the initial stages of acute pancreatitis, amylase levels may be normal during the recovery phase. An alternative is to measure the urine amylase level; however, even mild renal impairment may make interpretation of an elevated level difficult.

In an attempt to improve diagnostic accuracy, serum pancreatic lipase has been measured in conjunction with, or in place of, amylase but this does not add significantly to the diagnostic accuracy. Measurement of other pancreatic enzymes, such as trysinogen-2, may be useful in the early diagnosis of pancreatitis caused by endoscopic retrograde cholangiopancreatography (ERCP). However, in general, measuring serum amylase is not sufficiently specific or sensitive to be used as a diagnostic test in isolation. Liver function tests are important in diagnosing obstructive jaundice or cholangitis due to gallstones.

Table 12.1 – The Glasgow score. More than three criteria indicates severe pancreatitis (in 48 h).

Age	>55 years
WBC	$>15 \times 10^9\,l^{-1}$
Urea	$>16\,mmol.l^{-1}$
Arterial P_aO_2	$<8.0\,kPa$
Albumin	$<32\,g.l^{-1}$
Calcium	$<2.0\,mmol.l^{-1}$
Lactate dehydrogenase	$>600\,i.u.\cdot l^{-1}$
Aspartate aminotransferase	$>200\,i.u.\cdot l^{-1}$

Pancreatitis has effects on glucose metabolism, initiates the inflammatory response, increases vascular permeability and impairs organ function. A number of scoring systems, which utilise markers of these processes, can be used to assess the severity of illness and outcome. The most commonly used are the Glasgow (Table 12.1) and Ranson scores (Table 12.2). C-reactive protein is an easily measured (normal levels $<10\,mg.l^{-1}$) marker of disease activity. Sequential measures of organ function, such as the Sequential Organ Assessment Score, are available and may be useful for monitoring disease progression.

Table 12.2 – The Ranson score. A score $\geqslant 3$ indicates severe acute pancreatitis. One point is given for each criteria.

	Parameter
On admission	
Age	>55 years
WBC	$>16\,000.mm^{-3}$
Blood glucose	$>11.1\,mmol.l^{-1}$
Lactate dehydrogenase	$>350\,i.u.\cdot l^{-1}$
Aspartate aminotransferase	$>250\,i.u.\cdot l^{-1}$
During first 24 h	
Absolute decrease in haematocrit	>10%
Increase in urea	$>1.8\,mmol.l^{-1}$
Serum calcium	$<2\,mmol.l^{-1}$
Arterial P_aO_2	$<8.0\,kPa$
Base deficit	$>4\,mmol.l^{-1}$
Fluid sequestration	$>6\,l$

Radiological findings

Multi-organ involvement is common in severe pancreatitis. Patient outcome depends upon the severity of the pancreatic necrosis and the presence or absence of infectious complications. Radiology has a key role in assessing the severity of the attack and identifying the need for further diagnostic and therapeutic manoeuvres. Plain abdominal and chest films may demonstrate the following:

1. a localised ileus ('sentinel loop');

2. the 'colon cut-off' sign (due to local spasm);

3. a blurred psoas shadow (due to retroperitoneal pancreatic necrosis);

4. a raised hemidiaphragm;

5. plural effusion;

6. atelectasis; and

7. pulmonary infiltrates suggesting Acute Lung Injury or Acute Respiratory Distress Syndrome.

Abdominal ultrasound is of value in assessing the biliary tree for obstruction (gallstones are a leading cause of pancreatitis) and detecting peritoneal fluid collections. However, abdominal CT scanning is superior and should be used if patients with clinical or biochemical evidence of pancreatitis fail to respond to conservative therapy (Figure 12.1).

CT-guided aspiration and drainage of intra-abdominal fluid collections can be performed; microbiological analysis will aid the diagnosis of intra-abdominal infection. Areas of pancreatic necrosis are best identified using contrast-enhanced CT studies. The severity of the pancreatitis seen on CT can be graded using a scale from A to E as described by Balthazar (Table 12.3).

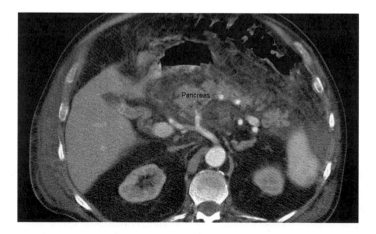

Figure 12.1 – A contrast-enhanced CT scan showing a normally enhancing pancreas (i.e. no necrosis) but extensive peri-pancreatic swelling and inflammation.

Table 12.3 – The Balthazar score. Unenhanced CT severity index score plus necrosis score. A maximum score of 10.

Grade		Score
On unenhanced CT scan		
A	Normal pancreas	0
B	Focal or diffuse enlargement	1
C	Peri-pancreatic inflammation with intrinsic pancreatic abnormalities	2
D	Intra- or extra-pancreatic fluid collections	3
E	Two or more large collections of gas, in pancreas or retroperitoneum	4
Necrosis score on contrast-enhanced CT (% necrosis)		
0		0
<33%		2
33–50%		4
>50%		6

When combined with an index of pancreatic necrosis, this score can be used to create a CT severity index for acute pancreatitis.

The aetiology of pancreatitis is often difficult to determine. It can broadly be divided into:

1. gallstones;

2. alcohol;

3. infection;

4. hypertriglyceridaemia;

5. others, including trauma, ERCP, malignancy, congenital abnormalities, inherited predisposition and hypercalcaemia; and

6. idiopathic.

Gallstones, particularly small stones or sludge, alcohol and infections are common aetiologies. Pancreatitis due to alcohol is more common in men, while that due to gallstones is more common in women. Viral infections due to mumps virus, coxsackie virus, *Cytomegalovirus*, *Varicella zoster* or *Herpes simplex* may occur at any age. Other infective causes include bacteria, fungi and parasites. Hypertriglyceridaemia may cause pancreatitis, especially in children. Hypercalcaemia may also provoke pancreatitis and there may be a link with hyperparathyroidism. Rare causes include malignancy, drugs, trauma, ERCP, pancreatic ischaemia and pregnancy. Approximately, one-third of patients have no identified cause and, in others, the presence of a risk factor may be coincidental rather than being the cause.

PATHOLOGY AND PATHOPHYSIOLOGY

The pancreas has important endocrine and exocrine functions. Therefore, pancreatic inflammation that causes a lack of insulin and the systemic release of digestive enzyme may have significant effects on both glucose homeostasis and digestion. Inflammation and oedema may also affect common bile duct drainage and the vascular supply to adjacent organs (e.g. spleen). Most, if not all, of the clinical deterioration seen in patients with pancreatitis is due to the systemic effects caused by activation of the inflammatory response. In addition, areas of pancreatic necrosis and intra-abdominal fluid collections can become infected.

The pathogenesis of acute pancreatitis is not fully understood. Different insults, such as long-term alcohol intake and gallstones, lead to a similar clinical picture, although the precipitants are clearly different. Irrespective of the trigger, pancreatic enzymes continue to be synthesised despite an inability for them to be secreted. Local pancreatic defence mechanisms are overwhelmed by a massive release of trypsin leading to pancreatic injury. Local release of inflammatory mediators (e.g. interleukins 1, 6 and 8), arachidonic acid metabolites, proteolytic enzymes and oxygen free radicals leads to systemic leucocyte activation, cytokine release and SIRS. Eventually, other organs fail causing acute respiratory distress, renal impairment and cardiovascular collapse. It is also postulated that gut mucosal barrier breakdown leads to translocation of bacteria from the gut lumen into the portal bloodstream and lymphatics, thereby increasing the risk of peritoneal infection.

THERAPEUTIC GOALS

The therapeutic goals in this patient include:

1. Establishing the correct diagnosis and removing triggering agents.

2. Resuscitation and general organ support are required until the pancreatitis resolves.

3. Definitive treatment of complications.

4. Prevention of recurrence.

THERAPEUTIC OPTIONS BASED ON PHYSIOLOGICAL AND PHARMACOLOGICAL EFFECTS

Resuscitation and maintenance of organ function

The general management of patients with severe pancreatitis is based upon simple intensive care measures. Fluid resuscitation, guided by invasive cardiovascular monitoring, may be required to restore circulating volume and to achieve adequate arterial perfusion pressure. Inotropic and vasopressor drugs may be required to improve cardiac output and to increase systemic vascular resistance. Despite adequate resuscitation, acute tubular necrosis may occur due to poor cardiac output, hypovolaemia or sepsis; dialysis or continuous haemofiltration may be required.

Respiratory support is frequently required because the acute respiratory distress syndrome is common in severe pancreatitis. In addition, abdominal swelling may be considerable, leading to splinting of the diaphragms. A ventilatory strategy that prevents airway closure, but minimises volutrauma, is required. Adequate levels of positive end-expiratory pressure and tidal volumes of around $6\,ml.kg^{-1}$ are thought to produce better outcomes than the higher tidal volumes previously used.

Nutrition

Continuous nasogastric feeding is now known to be safe in pancreatitis and is preferred to the parenteral route, which has a greater incidence of infective complications. Although nasojejunal feeding is the preferred route, nasogastric feeding has also been successfully used. Theoretical advantages of enteral feeding include reducing bacterial overgrowth, reducing translocation of bacteria and avoiding total parenteral nutrition related complications. A number of techniques are available to ensure correct placement of the nasojejunal tube but endoscopes ensure optimal positioning.

Prophylactic antibiotics

Although the infective complications of pancreatitis may be reduced with prophylactic antibiotics, there has been no reduction in sepsis related mortality. Furthermore, prophylactic antibiotics are associated with an increase in infections due to resistant organisms and fungi. At present, the administration of prophylactic antibiotics is controversial and no clear consensus exists.

Diagnosing and treating infection

Prompt treatment of cholangitis is essential; diagnosis is aided by liver function tests and an abdominal ultrasound scan to detect a dilated biliary tree. A jaundiced patient with gallstone pancreatitis needs an urgent ERCP and sphincterotomy; insertion of a common bile duct stent may also be required. Later in the disease course, infection of the necrotic pancreas or intra-abdominal fluid collections requires radiological or surgical drainage, together with antibiotic cover. Removal of the dead pancreatic tissue, often called necrosectomy, can be performed at laparotomy (Figure 12.2).

Post-operatively the pancreatic bed can be lavaged via large intra-abdominal drains to remove residual necrotic or infected tissue. Large volumes of fluid (up to $24\,l.day^{-1}$) are required for this technique; warmed renal dialysate fluid will minimise temperature and biochemical derangements.

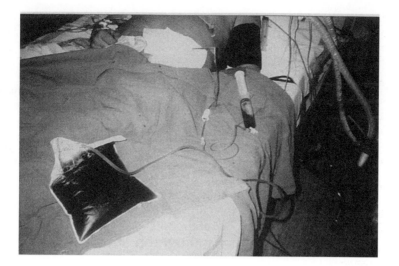

Figure 12.2 – Necrotic fluid draining from the pancreatic bed (reproduced with permission from Ryan DW, Park GR. *Color Atlas of Critical and Intensive Care*. London: Mosby-Wolfe, 1995:26).

Establishing cause and preventing recurrence

All cases of gallstone-related pancreatitis require a cholecystectomy. Avoidance of other triggering agents (e.g. alcohol) is desirable.

USUAL OUTCOME

The overall mortality rate for acute severe pancreatitis is between 20% and 30%. However, the outcome for the individual patient depends on the severity of the attack and, in particular, the degree of pancreatic necrosis. The inflammatory stimulus will determine the extent of multiple-organ dysfunction and patients frequently die as a result of sepsis. Pseudocysts may develop in the recovery phase and require surgical drainage. Exocrine insufficiency can be present in 80% of survivors and subclinical or insulin-dependent diabetes can develop in 50% of patients in the first 4 months following an attack, especially, if the patients have undergone surgery. Functional and anatomical abnormalities can persist for years but most tend to improve within a year after an acute attack.

KEY LEARNING POINTS

1. Abdominal pain, vomiting and elevated amylase levels are the principle diagnostic markers; CT scanning in the radiological investigation of choice for assessing the severity of the disease.

2. The commonest two causes of pancreatitis are alcohol abuse and gall-stones, account for 85% of cases in total.

3. Severity of the disease depends upon the magnitude of the inflammatory reaction occurring in the retroperitoneal space, whether pancreatic necrosis has occurred and, if bacterial infection has supervened.

4. Multiple-organ dysfunction results due to the release of inflammatory mediators, activated enzymes and vasoactive substances into the systemic circulation.

5. Mortality depends upon severity but overall is between 10% and 20%.

Further reading

1. Baron TH, Morgan DE. Acute necrotising pancreatitis. *New England Journal of Medicine* 1999; **340**: 1412–17.

2. Balthazar EJ, Robinson DL, Megibow AJ, Ranson JH. Acute pancreatitis; value of CT in establishing prognosis. *Radiology* 1990; **174**: 331–6.

3. Banks PA. Practice guidelines in acute pancreatitis. *American Journal of Gastroenterology* 1997; **92**: 377–86.

4. Corfield AP, Cooper MJ, Williamson RC *et al.* Prediction of severity in acute pancreatitis: prospective comparison of three prognostic indices. *Lancet* 1985; **2**: 403–7.

13

TRANSFER OF A CRITICALLY INJURED YOUNG TRAUMA VICTIM TO THE REGIONAL NEUROSURGICAL SERVICE

S Ridley

CASE SCENARIO

A previously fit, 21-year-old male is admitted to the intensive care unit (ICU), having been extricated from a road traffic accident 2 h earlier. His Glasgow Coma Scale (GCS) score on arrival is 6. One hour later, he has been intubated, paralysed and sedated and his circulation is stable. X-rays of the cervical spine are normal, and a CT scan of the head shows a small extradural haematoma and widespread scattered intra-cerebral contusions. The patient's chest X-ray suggests that he has broken seven ribs (three to nine inclusive) on the left. His clinical condition and CT scan have been reviewed over the telephone by the local regional neurosurgical service. It is felt that, while he may not need immediate operative intervention for his extradural haematoma, intra-cerebral pressure monitoring is indicated. The patient requires transfer to the neurosurgical centre 25 miles away.

DEFINITION AND DESCRIPTION OF THE PROBLEM

The aim is to prevent secondary brain damage, which may be caused by hypoxaemia, hypercapnia and hypotension, by thorough resuscitation and treatment prior to transfer and continued careful observation and monitoring throughout transfer.

The primary brain damage (occurring at the time of injury) has already caused neuronal loss. Secondary brain damage will compound the brain swelling associated with the primary injury and this will exacerbate rises in intra-cranial pressure (ICP). ICP monitoring will detect raised ICP, thereby allowing the use of treatments to minimise surges of pressure and optimise cerebral blood flow.

During movement, critically ill patients display adverse cardiorespiratory responses. Maintaining the standards of all aspects of care for the critically ill patient during transfer is the challenge for the accompanying medical and nursing staff. There may be a conflict of clinical needs; the patient may require urgent and rapid referral to the neurosurgeon, but time is required for thorough assessment, resuscitation and monitoring prior to transfer.

PATHOLOGY AND PATHOPHYSIOLOGY OF BRAIN DAMAGE

Primary brain damage occurs at the moment of injury and this neurological damage is irreversible; however, if brain contusion and haematoma (intra-cerebral, subdural and extradural) are managed effectively, then death and disability may be avoided.

Secondary brain damage results from oedema, ischaemia, cell necrosis, raised ICP and inadequate cerebral perfusion. At a cellular level, energy failure produced by inadequate oxygenation initiates a cascade of events that promote cell damage. These include increased levels of intra-cellular calcium, release of excitatory amino acids (especially glutamine), generation of free radicals such as superoxide (O_2^-), hydrogen peroxide (H_2O_2), hydroxyl (OH^-) and nitric oxide (NO). The cellular cytoskeleton and membrane breaks down, promoting further neuronal swelling and cell death.

Physiological response to brain injury

The pathological mechanisms of primary and secondary brain injury initiate a vicious cycle of physiological responses in the brain. The brain swells causing increased ICP, thus reducing cerebral blood flow. In turn, this contributes to further cellular ischaemia.

Brain oedema may be vasogenic or cytotoxic in origin. Vasogenic oedema is believed to occur soon after injury and results from cellular disruption of the blood brain barrier, allowing movement of protein-containing fluid into the interstitial space. Cytotoxic oedema occurs later and results from cellular swelling, secondary to the failure of energy generating pathways. These two types of oedema are not mutually exclusive, and usually brain swelling is maximal 24 or 48 h after injury.

ICP is determined by the volumes of cerebro-spinal fluid, blood and brain tissue within the skull; in the adult, the normal value for ICP is less than 15 mmHg. Once the usual compensatory mechanisms (i.e. reduced cerebro-spinal fluid and intra-cerebral blood volumes) are exhausted, an increase in brain tissue volume (due to swelling) will result in a precipitous increase in ICP. Sustained increases cause death due to brain herniation and brain stem compression. Less severe swelling leads to a reduction in cerebral blood flow and decreased oxygen delivery to the remaining functioning neurones, thereby exacerbating the injury.

Normal cerebral blood flow rate is approximately $50\,ml.100\,gm^{-1}.min^{-1}$. When the flow rate falls below $25\,ml.100\,gm^{-1}.min^{-1}$, electrical activity is lost. With a rate of $10\,ml.100\,gm^{-1}.min^{-1}$, cells are no longer capable of maintaining ionic homeostasis and cell death occurs. To deliver the optimum volumes of oxygen, cerebral blood flow is auto-regulated at perfusion pressures between 65 and 140 mmHg. Unfortunately, there is no simple bedside device for measuring cerebral blood flow, and cerebral perfusion pressure is a surrogate measure for blood flow.

Cerebral perfusion pressure is equal to mean arterial pressure minus ICP. In the head injured patient, the usual auto-regulatory mechanisms may be only partly or non-functioning. The auto-regulation curve of cerebral perfusion pressure may be moved to the right and a higher mean perfusion pressure (a minimum of 70–80 mmHg) is required to optimise cerebral blood flow. Outcome is significantly worse with cerebral perfusion pressures below 60 mmHg, and significantly better if the cerebral perfusion pressure has been maintained above 80 mmHg for the first 48 h.

THERAPEUTIC GOALS

The therapeutic goals dictate that:

1. The patient must be properly resuscitated making sure that the basic life supporting principles are observed.

2. The patient is prepared for transfer by thorough assessment, monitoring and further therapy, if required.

3. The aim of secondary transfer is to move a stable patient in an unhurried fashion between hospitals.

THERAPEUTIC OPTIONS BASED ON PHYSIOLOGICAL AND PHARMACOLOGICAL EFFECTS

A system-by-system approach is required to prepare the patient for transfer, and this can be combined with checks on the efficacy of basic life support measures.

Airway

For head injured patients, oral intubation is preferred because of the risk of further damage to the base of the skull, if the patient is intubated via the nose. The correct position of the tracheal tube should be checked radiographically. Once the correct position is confirmed, the tracheal tube should be securely attached to the patient so that it will neither move during transfer nor obstruct venous return from the head. Securing the tracheal tube at the mouth with adhesive tape is probably the most appropriate method of attachment.

It is impossible to over-emphasise the importance of cervical spine immobilisation. Normal plain cervical X-rays in an unconscious patient do not exclude a cervical injury. Only if the patient has undergone detailed CT examination of the whole cervical spine, can a serious bony injury be excluded. Therefore, in most situations, it is wise to leave the hard restraining cervical collar in place during transfer. The collar should be checked to see if it is the correct size for the patient and has been applied properly.

Breathing

When the patient is intubated and ventilated, the adequacy of gas exchange should be checked. The respiratory system should be examined both clinically and radiologically; the chest X-ray that was apparently normal in the Accident and Emergency Department may no longer be so, as the patient could have developed a tension pneumothorax, large haemothorax, ruptured diaphragm or pulmonary contusion. All of these need to be excluded or, if present, managed prior to transfer. As this patient has broken seven ribs, a chest drain inserted prior to transfer may avoid the development of a pneumothorax in transit.

The patient must be given neuromuscular blocking agents and sedatives, as coughing on the tracheal tube will further increase ICP. Sedation is humane and also reduces the cerebral metabolic requirement for oxygen, thereby preserving neuronal structure and function. If there is evidence of seizures, these need to be controlled prior to paralysis. Lorazepam is the drug of choice in the short term, but phenytoin ($15\,mg.kg^{-1}$) may also be required for longer term control.

In the ICU, the patient is ventilated by a sophisticated ventilator, but during transfer the ventilatory options will be fewer. Therefore, the patient should be attached to the transport ventilator with the settings adjusted to emulate the ventilatory pattern of the ICU ventilator. The adequacy of ventilation should then be checked clinically and by blood gas analysis after approximately 20 min.

Hypocapnia is a potent vaso-constrictor and may reduce ICP by reducing cerebral blood flow; however, hyperventilation must not be excessive as levels of P_aCO_2 less than 3.5 kPa promote ischaemic injury. Ideally, the transport ventilator should be adjusted to maintain P_aCO_2 between 4 and 4.5 kPa.

The choice of inspired oxygen tensions available on transport ventilators may be limited. When *en route*, haemodynamic changes may exacerbate ventilation–perfusion mismatch, so that the patient may become hypoxaemic if the F_iO_2 has not been set sufficiently high. If the transfer is lengthy, pathological processes which were not apparent in the ICU, for example, pulmonary contusion or neurogenic pulmonary oedema, may develop *en route*. For these reasons, the F_iO_2 during transfer should be set 20–30% higher than that used in the ICU. This poses little risk of oxygen toxicity.

Circulation

Haemodynamic stability is an absolute prerequisite prior to transfer. In young patients, compensatory mechanisms are very effective at masking hypovolaemia, such that hypotension is a late sign of circulatory compromise. Better indicators of hypovolaemia are cold peripheries, delayed capillary refill time, inadequate urine output and a pulse pressure that fluctuates with respiration. Scalp bleeding rarely causes hypovolaemia. Alternative causes of hypovolaemia must be sought, as the presence of lower rib fractures suggests splenic damage.

Hypovolaemia can be corrected with transfusion of red cells, colloids (e.g. starches) or crystalloids. Dextrose containing solutions should be avoided as water overload and hyperglycaemia exacerbate brain injury.

As this patient has left-side chest injuries, myocardial contusion and pericardial tamponade could be the cause of hypotension. If pericardial tamponade is suspected, then echocardiography should be performed.

Invasive monitoring of the cardiovascular system is essential during transfer. Motion artefacts may render non-invasive blood pressure methods unreliable; direct intra-arterial measurement of blood pressure is preferable. Central venous access helps guide fluid resuscitation and provides reliable venous access for drug infusion and administration while en route. If the cause of the haemodynamic instability is unclear, a pulmonary artery catheter or oesophageal Doppler probe may be inserted prior to transfer. However, if a pulmonary artery catheter is inserted, the pulmonary artery trace must be displayed continuously during transfer to allow detection of inadvertent wedging; if the trace cannot be displayed, the catheter should be pulled back into the right atrium or superior vena cava.

The patient must be normovolaemic, and preferably hypervolaemic, prior to transfer. Critically ill patients display a variety of haemodynamic responses to movement. These include hypertension and tachycardia (caused by inadequate sedation) or, more commonly, hypotension and bradycardia (caused by peripheral vasodilatation and pooling of blood). As the sympathetic nervous system vascular control mechanisms have been obtunded by injury or sedation, pooling of blood may occur in response to the acceleration or deceleration forces experienced during transfer.

The electrocardiogram (ECG), end-tidal CO_2 and peripheral arterial oxygen saturation should also be continuously displayed on the transport monitor.

Essential equipment

A large amount of equipment is required to ensure that the patient can be moved safely; it may be divided into four broad categories. The first is that needed for basic care, such as the ICU bed or cot, laundry, sources of warmth and comfort.

Life support equipment such as the ventilator and other respiratory support, including oxygen supply may be considered as the second category; most of this will already have been attached to the patient during stabilisation on ICU. Monitoring devices and equipment required to treat the patient form the last two categories. Treatment equipment may be subdivided into that needed for continuing intensive therapy and that required in sudden physiological deterioration or equipment failure, such as a blocked tracheal tube, loss of oxygen, power failure and disconnected intravenous infusion lines. This equipment must be carried in anticipation of problems *en route* and its presence should be confirmed before transfer (Table 13.1). However,

Table 13.1 – Equipment template.

(a) Life support

Airway

Laryngoscopes, spare batteries and bulbs	Sterile-cuffed tracheal tubes (various sizes)
Sterile-cuffed tracheotomy tubes (various sizes)	Tracheal tube introducers (metal and gum elastic)
Catheter mounts	Tape and adhesive dressing
Disposable humidifiers	Magill forceps
Fixed performance oxygen masks and piping	Airways, oral and nasal (various sizes)
Lubricating jelly	Suction catheters and suction device
Artery forceps	

Breathing

Portable ventilators, ideally capable of volume-controlled ventilation, positive-end expiratory pressure generation and variable inspired oxygen fraction; Lightweight, simple, gas driven, robust and reliable	Oxygen cylinder with appropriate pressure reducing valves for ventilator and fresh gas flow to facemask
Disposable (or autoclavable) ventilator tubing	Self-inflating resuscitation bag with anaesthetic masks (various sizes)

Circulation

Intravenous cannulae (various sizes)	Central venous catheters (various lengths and diameters)
Cannulae appropriate for intra-arterial pressure monitoring	Sutures and dressings
Intravenous fluids and administration sets	Infusion pumps with appropriate syringes
Three-way luer lock taps and intravenous line extensions	

(b) Emergencies: Emergency drugs (in addition to those required as part of the ICU therapy)

Miscellaneous

Naso-gastric tubes (various sizes)	Scissors and razors
Syringes/needles	Sterile plain and alcohol-soaked swabs
Gloves and aprons	Documentation for transfer and the patient's medical notes

Mandatory extras (inter-hospital transfer) and optional extras (which should be easily available from elsewhere in the hospital)

Chest drains with Heimlich valves or underwater drains	DC defibrillator
	Anaeroid sphygmomanometer
Disposable pressure transducers and pressure infusion bags should be connected to the patient prior to transfer	Blood filters

it is important to emphasise that if pre-transfer stabilisation is performed properly, little of this equipment should be required.

Mannitol should be taken in case there are signs of neurological deterioration (e.g. pupillary changes) during transfer. It should be given rapidly (over 20 min) in the dose of $0.5 \, \text{gm.kg}^{-1}$ to reduce ICP. Mannitol has various effects; its immediate effect on ICP is ascribed to its improving blood rheology. It also acts as a volume expander, so improving cerebral blood flow, and as an osmotic diuretic helping to remove extra-vascular water from the brain.

Final checks

Just prior to departure, a checklist, such as that prepared by the Intensive Care Society (Table 13.2), should be reviewed. In addition, checks should confirm that:

1. all intravascular lines and other catheters or drains are well secured for transfer;

Table 13.2 – Is your patient ready for transfer?

Departure checklist
Attendants
Adequately experienced?
Knowledge of this case?
Clothed?
Insured?
Appropriate equipment and drugs?
Batteries checked?
Sufficient oxygen?
Trolley available?
Ambulance service aware/ready?
Bed confirmed?
Exact location?
Case notes, X-rays, results and blood collected?
Transfer chart prepared?
Portable phone charged?
Contact numbers known?
Money/cards for emergencies?
Estimated time of arrival notified?
Return arrangements checked?
Relatives informed?
Patient stable and fully investigated?
Monitoring attached? Functioning?
Drugs, pumps and lines rationalised/secured?
Adequate sedation?
Still stable after transfer to mobile equipment?
Anything missed?

2. the patient has received tetanus toxoid injection, where appropriate;

3. an oro-gastric tube has been passed;

4. gravity feed lines have been replaced with appropriate infusion pumps with either adequate battery life or replacement power sources;

5. the patient is being nursed slightly head up; and

6. the patient remains stable.

USUAL OUTCOME

The desired end point prior to departure is a well-resuscitated normo- or even hypervolaemic intubated and sedated patient, who has the important physiological variables (i.e. intra-arterial blood pressure, ECG, end-tidal CO_2 and peripheral arterial oxygen saturation) normalised and monitored and who has had all other injuries excluded or appropriately managed. Transfers that are undertaken properly will have few complications directly attributable to the transfer itself. Reports of complications during transfer (e.g. hypotension, hypoxaemia, missed injuries and hypothermia) are now rare, as these dangers have been recognised. In the UK, over 11 000 patients are transferred between critical care units annually and now most complete their journey safely.

KEY LEARNING POINTS

1. Transfer is inherently dangerous for the patient. There are well-recognised physiological responses to transfer and these should be anticipated.

2. All patients will require thorough assessment, resuscitation and monitoring to ensure their airway is protected, respiratory function is supported and that they are cardiovascularly stable and well filled.

3. It is vital to appreciate that while *en route* no further interventions are feasible because of the adverse environmental conditions and, therefore, anything that should be done must be done prior to departure. If anything needs to be done while moving, the safest option is to stop the ambulance before carrying out any interventions.

4. Checklists for equipment and physiological status prior to transfer have been published. These should be followed.

5. The ultimate aim is to move a stable patient in a timely, but unhurried fashion to the appropriate neurosurgical referral centre.

Further reading

1. Morton NS, Pollack MM, Wallace PGM. *Stabilization and Transport of the Critically Ill.* New York: Churchill Livingstone, 1997.

2. Wallace PGM, Ridley SA. Transport of critically ill patients. In Singer M, Grant I (eds), *ABC of Intensive Care.* London: BMJ Publishing, 1999: 39–42.

3. Intensive Care Society. *Guidelines for Transport of the Critically Ill Adult.* London: Intensive Care Society, 2002.

4. Association of Anaesthetists of Great Britain and Ireland. *Recommendations for the Transfer of Patients with Acute Head Injuries to Neurosurgical Units.* London: Association of Anaesthetists of Great Britain and Ireland, 1996.

5. Runcie CJ, Reeve WR, Wallace PG. Preparation of the critically ill for inter-hospital transfer. *Anaesthesia* 1992; **47**: 327–31.

6. Ridley SA. Secondary transport of the critically ill. *Anaesthesia and Intensive Care Medicine* 2000; **1**: 102–4.

7. Webb AR, Shapiro MJ, Singer M, Suter PM. *Oxford Textbook of Critical Care.* Oxford: Oxford Medical Publications, 1999: 820–35.

14

BURNS FOLLOWING AN ELECTRICAL FIRE IN AN ENCLOSED SPACE

A Batchelor

CASE SCENARIO

A 35-year-old male is admitted to the Accident and Emergency (A&E) Department after having been rescued from a smoke-filled room by firemen wearing breathing apparatus. He is an electrical contractor and the cause of the fire may have been electrical. On arrival at A&E, approximately 45 min after the rescue, he remains unconscious with a Glasgow Coma Scale (GCS) score of 5. The patient has extensive burns covering about 60% of his body surface area (BSA) including his face. He has a tachycardia (120 beats.min^{-1}) and is tachypnoeic (25 breaths.min^{-1}). No other history is available.

DEFINITION AND DESCRIPTION OF THE PROBLEM

The majority of burns occur in the home and are the result of carelessness and accidents; however, assault is occasionally involved. Outcome from major burns is related to the size and depth of burn, age (being worst at the extremes of age), and presence of inhalational injury. Major burns are those exceeding 25% BSA in adults, 20% at the extremes of age or 10% if the burns are full thickness. The presence of facial or neck burns, inhalational injury, associated trauma or significant co-morbidities will convert a smaller BSA burn into a major burn. Burns can be caused by flame, scald, electricity or chemicals. There may be co-incidental pathology such as fractures or internal bleeding; it is important to obtain as much information as possible about the mechanism of injury.

The outcome from major burns has improved significantly over the past 40 years. Small burns have always been associated with a low risk of death, and large burns in elderly people with a high mortality rate. In the USA, where data has been collected for a number of years on large numbers of patients, the greatest difference in outcome is in young adults with large burns in whom mortality has been reduced by 50% between the 1950s and late 1980s. This reduction has been associated with changes in practice including early resuscitation, better infection control, topical anti-microbials, early and better surgical treatment and better understanding and management of inhalation injury.

Airway swelling can be life threatening, and the airway must be secured early if there are facial or neck burns. Burn injury causes a systemic inflammatory response affecting all organ systems. The stress response to injury leads to excessive catabolism, weight loss, muscle wasting, reduced healing and affects the immune response. Temperature control is also impaired.

Patients with major burns require admission to a specialised critical care facility (e.g. a burn unit or its associated intensive care unit (ICU)). Patients with facial and airway burns or suspected or proven inhalational injury should be managed in an ICU.

PATHOLOGY AND PATHOPHYSIOLOGY OF BURNS

Burn injury produces both local and systemic responses. The local injury consists of three areas, the central zone of coagulative necrosis, an intermediate area of ischaemia and an outer ring of hyperaemia. The ischaemic zone is viable, but the precariously perfused tissue is vulnerable to necrosis, if resuscitation is inadequate or there is subsequent tissue oedema. The zone of hyperaemia produces inflammatory mediators and local vasodilatation. In patients with a total burn exceeding 25% BSA, this leads to capillary leak and albumin loss similar to that seen in systemic sepsis. In addition, fluid and albumin are lost directly from damaged skin. These losses lead to hypovolaemia. Fluid resuscitation is essential, but it can lead to tissue oedema severe enough to produce airway obstruction, cerebral oedema or abdominal compartment syndrome. Oedema worsens tissue hypoxia and may lead to organ failure involving the lungs, kidneys and gut. Myocardial contractility is also impaired by myocardial depressant factors at the very time that increased tissue oxygenation is required.

Depth of burn

The depth of burn determines whether the burn will heal spontaneously or whether excision and skin grafting will be required. The depth of burn can be divided into the following.

Superficial burns

Superficial burns can be further sub-divided into epithelial and superficial dermal. Both are intensely painful, as the nerve endings are damaged but not destroyed. Epithelial burns heal rapidly; a typical example is sunburn. Epithelial burns should not be included in the total area of burn for fluid calculations. Superficial dermal burns cause damage down to the upper part of the dermis. However, the presence of islands of epithelium in hair follicles and sweat glands permit healing without intervention. Superficial dermal burns are associated with blisters (i.e. a roof of dead skin containing fluid from the tissues beneath). The dermis beneath the blister is vulnerable to further injury.

Deep burns

Deep burns are either deep dermal or full thickness; both require excision and skin grafting to heal. Neither type is painful because the nerve endings are destroyed. Deep dermal burns are also associated with blister formation. The base of the blister is red and shows no capillary refill because the capillaries have been destroyed. Full thickness burns involve damage not only of both layers of the skin, but also fat and the structures beneath. They appear white and leathery and have no capillary refill.

Circumferential burns of limbs or digits may result in distal ischaemia as tissue oedema forms or the burn injury contracts. Circumferential burns of the chest and abdomen will impair respiration and perfusion to intra-abdominal organs. In such cases, escharotomy, an incision down to unburnt tissue, may be required.

Airway burns

Inhalational injury may cause airway burns or poisoning with noxious substances (e.g. carbon monoxide and hydrogen cyanide). Inhalation injuries increase mortality by 20–40% compared to an uncomplicated burn. Fluid requirements are increased by up to 50% in patients with inhalation injuries.

Airway burns occur because

1. the inhalation of hot gases burns the upper airway,

2. the lower airway is damaged by chemicals formed when noxious gases dissolve in water in the airway,

3. inhaled soot causes chemical damage to the airway mucosa.

Carbon monoxide inhalation may also impair oxygen delivery because carbon monoxide

1. has an affinity for haemoglobin 240 times that of oxygen;

2. combines with haemoglobin to form carboxyhaemoglobin, reducing the blood's ability to carry oxygen;

3. shifts the oxyhaemoglobin dissociation curve to the left, impairing tissue unloading of oxygen;

4. binds to myoglobin and cytochromes, making it difficult for tissues to utilise the available oxygen.

Cyanide is produced from burning plastics, such as polyurethane, and also inhibits oxygen delivery to the cells by inhibiting cytochrome oxidase and the tricarboxylic acid cycle, so that neither oxygen can be used nor adenosine triphosphate generated. The consequent anaerobic metabolism results in metabolic acidosis and high lactate levels.

Electrical burns

Electricity produces thermal burns by the generation of local heat. Electrical burns can be categorised as low or high tension, depending on the voltage. Low tension injuries are caused by voltages below 1000 V (e.g. household voltage). Alternating electrical current induces muscle spasm which may prolong exposure to the current. Low voltage is sufficient to cause cardiac arrest. High tension electrical burns include flash burns and injuries due to current transmission. If the current does not pass through the victim, but ignites clothing, simple thermal skin burns result. Current transmission through tissue produces entrance and exit wounds with tissue damage along its path. Internal damage may be much greater than is initially apparent from the skin wounds. Heating, caused by the resistance of tissues to the passage of current, causes swelling of muscle and can result in compartment syndrome, myoglobinuria and renal failure. Fasciotomies and, occasionally, amputation may be necessary. Hyperkalaemia, as a result of tissue necrosis, can be severe and should be expected.

Chemical burns (e.g. hydrofluric acid and phenol) are usually industrial injuries and health care workers need protective clothing to avoid contamination. Unlike flame burns, where removal from the fire prevents further injury, chemical burns can continue to cause damage until the agent is inactivated or removed. Hydrofluric acid is a particularly dangerous agent and can be fatal with as little as 2% BSA burn.

Pathophysiological response

The stress response to a major burn results in extensive catabolism of lean body tissue and weight loss, which contribute to morbidity and mortality. Early enteral nutrition is advocated. Gastric mucosal ulceration and bleeding is common and, therefore, mucosal protection using H_2-receptor antagonists should take place until full enteral feeding is tolerated.

Temperature control is lost after damage to large areas of the body surface. Essential, initial irrigation of burns with water that cools and limits burn injury may result in core cooling. Exposing the patient to permit full examination and assessment, and delay while transfer to the regional burns unit is arranged, can both result in further cooling. Cooling should be avoided as far as possible as the outcome is worse in hypothermic patients. After this initial period, pyrexia is common.

Infection is a major cause of death in patients with major burns. However, there is no indication for prophylactic antibiotics and infections should be treated as they arise. Tetanus prophylaxis may be needed.

Burns may be very painful, and pain relief is a challenge throughout the stay in critical care. Functional outcome may not be good from extensive burns and psychological support is essential.

THERAPEUTIC GOALS

The therapeutic goals in a patient with a severe burn include:

1. Adequate resuscitation to restore circulating volume without exacerbating oedema.

2. Support of organ function.

3. Microbiological surveillance with prompt treatment of infection.

4. Reduction of catabolism and the provision of nutrition.

5. Return to an independent lifestyle with the minimum possible residual deficit.

THERAPEUTIC OPTIONS BASED ON PHYSIOLOGICAL AND PHARMACOLOGICAL EFFECTS

Airway

Local burns to the face, neck, mouth and nose, singeing of nasal hairs or a hoarse voice are indications for intubation. A patient, whose airway looks unremarkable at first, can rapidly become difficult or impossible to intubate once oedema accumulates. A GCS lesser than 9 is also an indication for intubation.

Breathing

A patient with isolated facial burns and no history of inhalation injury may be able and permitted to breathe spontaneously on either a T-piece or a continuous positive airway pressure (CPAP) circuit after the airway is secured by tracheal intubation. Patients with more severe injuries should be ventilated to ensure adequate gas exchange. If there is a suspicion of carbon monoxide inhalation or the patient has been unconscious, 100% oxygen should be administered until the results of carboxyhaemoglobin levels are obtained and are known to have declined to less than 5%. Hyperbaric oxygen is difficult to administer in the acute phase of resuscitation and there are few centres capable of its administration; its use remains controversial.

Cyanide poisoning is difficult to diagnose but should be suspected if inhalational injury is likely and the patient has high carboxyhaemoglobin levels. Usually cyanide poisoning can be treated with oxygen and ventilation; however, thiosulphate could be given to enhance hepatic conversion of cyanide to thiocyanate. Sodium nitrite can be given to produce methaemoglobin which combines with cyanide to produce cyanmethaemoglobin; however, neither of these compounds carry oxygen. Therefore, in a patient who also has carbon monoxide poisoning, the reduction in oxygen transport could be critical and so sodium nitrite should be used carefully.

Circumferential burns of the thorax may require escharotomies to permit ventilation; diagrams illustrating suitable incision sites can be faxed from burns units, if there is no appropriately trained person available. Incisions are made down to bleeding tissue. In the presence of a severe burn, the acute respiratory distress syndrome (ARDS) is likely to develop, especially if there is an associated inhalational injury. For those patients who will require long-term respiratory support, early tracheostomy is indicated. In some patients with burns of the neck, it may be appropriate to graft the front of the neck early to permit tracheostomy.

Circulation

Two large peripheral cannulae should be inserted, preferably through non-burnt tissue. Fluid requirements can be calculated using the Parkland formula (i.e. 3–4 ml.kg^{-1}.% burn^{-1} of Hartmanns solution to be administered in the 24 h from the time of injury). Half is given in the first 8 h, the remainder in the following 16 h). In patients with extensive burns, assessment of adequacy of resuscitation can be difficult and invasive monitoring of blood pressure is essential. Central venous line insertion is advisable for both monitoring and drug administration purposes. Where possible, catheters should be sited through unburned skin. Other guides to the adequacy of fluid replacement include the urine output (>0.5–1 ml.kg^{-1}.h^{-1}) and the peripheral perfusion of unburnt tissue. In the absence of carbon monoxide or cyanide poisoning, a persistent acidosis is likely to represent inadequate fluid replacement. The Parkland formula should be regarded as a rough guide to fluid requirements; significantly more fluid than calculated may be needed. The normal hourly maintenance fluid must be given in addition to that calculated for the burn losses. Calculation of area of burned skin is assessed using the 'Rule of 9s'. The body surface is divided into 11 areas, each of which covers approximately 9% BSA (Figure 14.1).

After the initial 24 h, fluid requirements remain high. Opinion is divided as to the relative benefits of crystalloids or colloids; if colloid is used, hydroxyethyl starch should be considered. The role of albumin is unclear and in many units, its use has been discontinued. While it is desirable to avoid excessive oedema, it is vitally important to ensure adequate resuscitation as early as possible after the injury. As a result, it may be necessary to accept a degree of unavoidable swelling. As in sepsis,

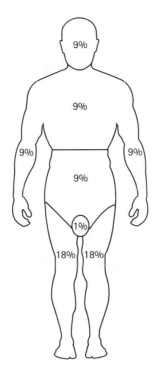

Figure 14.1 – The 'Rule of 9s' whereby the adult BSA is broken down in areas of 9%, 18% and 1%.

vasopressors (e.g. norepinephrine) may be required to maintain an adequate perfusion pressure, but should only be administered once it is certain that sufficient fluid has been given. Even after a period of stability, essential surgery may result in a further period of circulatory instability.

If there is a history of electrical injury, an electrocardiogram (ECG) should be performed to exclude myocardial damage. An elevation of the cardiac enzyme, Troponin I, is associated with the myocardial depression seen with major burns even in the absence of direct myocardial damage. Renal failure is associated with an increase in mortality and resuscitation should be aimed at preventing its occurrence. If the patient has myoglobinuria, a higher hourly urine output ($>1\,\mathrm{ml.kg^{-1}.h^{-1}}$) should be maintained.

Nutrition

Starting enteral nutrition within the first 24 h is possible in most patients with burns; if gastric emptying is delayed, a naso–jejunal tube should be placed. Total parenteral nutrition increases the incidence of infectious complications and should be reserved for those patients in whom enteral feeding is impossible. Interruptions in feeding should be kept to a minimum; for instance, it is unnecessary to 'starve' an intubated patient prior to theatre. The bowel mucosa derives a proportion of its metabolic requirements from the bowel lumen, so by starting enteral feeding early, it may be possible to maintain gut mucosal integrity. The best defence against stress ulceration is enteral feeding. Nutritional requirements are higher than normal and skilled dietetic input is helpful. Daily protein requirement may be estimated as $1 \text{g.kg}^{-1} + 3 \text{g.}\%BSA$; 20% of the kilocalories should be protein and the non-protein calorie-to-nitrogen ratio decreased to 100:1. Trace elements including copper, zinc and selenium are particularly depleted and this results in poor outcomes; these should be replaced, if necessary intravenously, and levels should be checked frequently.

Infection

The major cause of mortality in patients with burns is infection. Attention to cleanliness, especially hand-washing, is paramount. Early debridement and grafting results in protection of the zone of ischaemia and prevents further local damage; infection can destroy the grafts and in patients with limited donor sites, it may be weeks before skin cover can be replaced. Burned patients have impaired immunity because their skin barrier has been lost. Invasive devices (e.g. catheters, tubes, drains) are portals for infection; regular cultures should be taken from these as well as burn sites.

Other injuries

The presence of large burns can easily distract attention from other significant injuries. Unconsciousness could be due to carbon monoxide poisoning, epilepsy or a head injury. A patient rescued from a road traffic accident may have multiple trauma as well as burns. Standard trauma protocols should be followed and patients should be admitted to hospital via the A&E Department, to facilitate full examination and assessment and not directly to the burns unit.

Temperature

On admission to hospital, patients are frequently hypothermic. Re-warming should be cautious and proceed in tandem with fluid resuscitation. After re-warming, it is common for the patient's temperature to rise above normal. Temperatures exceeding 40°C should be reduced actively by the removal of burns dressings, or the use of fans, paracetamol, gastric lavage or extracorporeal circulation. Temperatures in excess of 42°C may result in cerebral injury.

Pain relief

Superficial burns and skin donor sites are intensely painful. In the acute phase, the patient will receive intravenous sedation and analgesia. In the recovery phase, when the patient is awake, opiates, ketamine, tricyclic antidepressants, non-steroidal anti-inflammatory drugs and anticonvulsant agents may be useful. Anaesthesia may still be required for dressing changes.

Surgery

Patients with major burns require frequent surgery. Each trip to the operating theatre requires the same amount of organisation and preparation as a transfer to another hospital. Debridement of large areas of burn, followed by the removal of skin for grafting, can result in major blood loss. Large bore venous access and rapid transfusion devices may be needed. Each episode of surgery is a new systemic insult to an already compromised patient, and may result in a temporary requirement for cardiovascular support. The timing of surgery should be decided jointly between intensivists, anaesthetists and surgeons. Specific burn sites need different management. For example, buttock burns may be difficult to keep clean and grafts may be lost as a result. A temporary defunctioning stoma may be required, and early skin grafting to an area of abdominal wall may be necessary to permit this. Vascular access can become a problem and grafting over the jugular, subclavian and femoral veins will be useful.

Psychological support

Major burns can be associated with significant loss of function and disfigurement; the patient may not be able to return to their previous activities and life-style. Psychological support should be started in the ICU.

Rehabilitation

Even while patients are critically ill, their rehabilitation needs to be considered. Physiotherapy to limbs is important, as muscle contractures and joint ankylosis rapidly occur in critically ill patients.

Team work

A successful outcome from major burns requires teamwork between intensivists, anaesthetists, plastic surgeons, nurses, physiotherapists, dieticians and psychologists. Patients should be referred early to a suitable burns facility.

USUAL OUTCOME

The mortality caused by burn injury is difficult to predict at presentation to the A&E Department. Undoubtedly, mortality is related to the depth of the burn, the BSA involved and the age of the patient. However, with improvements in burn management, mortality rates have fallen. Forty years ago, a young adult aged 30 with 50% BSA severe burns would have died. Today, the expected mortality of such a patient would be about 10%. Patients with the most severe burn (70–90%) now have mortality rates of about 50%. Previous estimates of mortality in burns victims (e.g. mortality = BSA burnt + age) are no longer accurate. The main cause of mortality in burn victims on ICU is infective complications, which cannot be predicted at presentation. If patients survive the physical insult of the burn, then psychological consequences will be more prominent.

KEY LEARNING POINTS

1. Beware of facial burns and inhalation injury. If in doubt, protect the airway by tracheal intubation.

2. Adequate fluid resuscitation is essential; crystalloid is the fluid of choice for the first 24 h.

3. Associated injuries must be excluded.

4. Treatment with vasoconstricting agents should only be commenced once adequate fluid resuscitation has been administered.

5. Enteral nutrition should be started as early as possible and interruptions kept to a minimum.

6. Antibiotics should not be used prophylactically, particularly, in the early phase of treatment.

7. Infection is life threatening. By restricting antibiotic use to narrow spectrum agents in short courses, the emergence of resistant infections may be limited or delayed.

8. Careful planning of the exact sequence of skin grafting requires a team discussion.

9. Pain relief can be difficult and involvement of the acute and chronic pain teams may be useful.

10. A major burn results in long-term disability. The ICU should be regarded as the first part of the rehabilitation process.

11. Team work is essential for a successful outcome.

Further reading

1. Australia and New Zealand Burn Association. *Emergency Management of Severe Burns, Course Manual.* Kelvin Grove, Queensland: Australia and New Zealand Burn Association Ltd, 1996.

2. Gueugniaud PY, Carsin H, Bertin-Maghit M, Petit P. Current advance in the initial management of major thermal burns. *Intensive Care Medicine* 2000; **26**: 848–56.

3. Pruitt BA. Protection from excessive resuscitation 'Pushing the pendulum back.' *Journal of Trauma* 2000; **49**: 567–8.

4. Raff T, Germann G, Hartmann B. The value of early enteral nutrition in the prophylaxis of stress ulceration in the severely burned patient. *Burns* 1997; **23**: 313–8.

5. Platt AJ, Aslam S, Judkins K. Temperature profiles during resuscitation predict survival following burns complicated by smoke. *Burns* 1997; **23**: 250–5.

6. Scheinkastel CD, Bailey M, Myles PS *et al.* Hyperbaric or normobaric oxygen for acute carbon monoxide poisoning: a randomised controlled clinical trial. *Medical Journal of Australia* 1999; **170**: 203–10.

7. Lorente JA, Ezpelata A, Esteban A *et al.* Systemic hemodynamics, gastric intra-mucosal PCO_2 changes and outcome in critically ill burn patients. *Critical Care Medicine* 2000; **28**: 1728–35.

8. Kaups KL, Davis JW, Dominic WJ. Base deficit as an indicator of resuscitation needs in patients with burn injuries. *Journal of Burn Care and Rehabilitation* 1998; **19**: 346–8.

9. Gore DC, Dalton JM, Gehr TWB. Colloid infusions reduce glomerular filtration in resuscitated burn victims. *Journal of Trauma* 1996; **40**: 356–60.

10. Murphy JT, Horton JW, Purdue GF, Hunt JL. Evaluation of Troponin I as an indicator of cardiac dysfunction after thermal injury. *Journal of Trauma* 1998; **45**: 700–4.

15

VENTILATORY FAILURE DUE TO MUSCLE WEAKNESS

B L Taylor

CASE SCENARIO

A previously fit, 74-year-old man with a 7-day history of dysphagia is referred for intensive care assessment because of an increasing oxygen requirement and progressive tachypnoea. He has recently recovered from an upper respiratory tract infection, which developed after he had spent Christmas with his grandchildren. He normally takes bendrofluazide and enalapril for hypertension.

When examined on the ward he has a respiratory rate of 45 breaths.min^{-1}, and a peripheral oxygen saturation of 93% on high flow oxygen. His arterial blood pressure is 90/45 mmHg, with a regular pulse rate of 65 beats.min^{-1}. He has an axillary temperature of 35.4°C. Ausculation of the chest reveals signs of a right basal pneumonia. Bedside testing reveals a vital capacity (VC) of 400 ml. He is drowsy, but opens his eyes to voice. He tries to move to command, but is globally weak and his speech is slurred. His deep tendon reflexes are absent in all limbs; he has a poor cough and is unable to swallow saliva. There is no evidence of muscle or tongue fasciculation. Direct questioning reveals that he has diminished sensation in both legs and in the tips of fingers on both hands. He also has double vision on lateral gaze.

Initial investigations are normal except for the white cell count ($26 \times 10^9 \mathrm{l}^{-1}$), urea ($15 \,\mathrm{mmol.l}^{-1}$) and creatinine ($180 \,\mu\mathrm{mol.l}^{-1}$). Arterial blood gases taken on high flow oxygen reveal a pH 7.26, P_aO_2 7.5 kPa, P_aCO_2 8.2 kPa, standard bicarbonate $18 \,\mathrm{mmol.l}^{-1}$ and a base excess $-8 \,\mathrm{mmol.l}^{-1}$.

DEFINITION AND DESCRIPTION OF THE PROBLEM

The patient has peripheral neurological failure, leading to immobility and global muscle weakness. Associated bulbar dysfunction has caused aspiration of pharyngeal contents leading to pneumonia. He has progressive ventilatory failure with retention of carbon dioxide. The presence of hypoxaemia, despite high flow oxygen, indicates that the combination of pneumonia, poor cough and respiratory muscle weakness have reduced his respiratory reserve.

The presence of hypotension may be secondary to a sepsis related inflammatory response or hypovolaemia, but the relative bradycardia and hypothermia suggest that there is also autonomic dysfunction. The history of a recent probable viral illness, with subsequent gradual weakness, bulbar dysfunction and paraesthesia suggests a diagnosis of acute post-infective polyneuropathy (i.e. Guillain–Barré syndrome).

Additional problems during long-term immobility are likely to include damage to pressure areas, risk of deep venous thrombosis, severe muscle wasting, psychological illness and critical care polyneuropathy.

PHYSIOLOGY AND PATHOPHYSIOLOGY OF GUILLAIN–BARRÉ SYNDROME

Guillain–Barré syndrome is a progressive demyelinating polyneuropathy which characteristically develops 2–3 weeks after an acute respiratory or gastrointestinal infection with micro-organisms such as *Campylobacter* or *Mycoplasma*. However, 10% of cases follow a recent surgical procedure; immunisation and streptokinase therapy have also been implicated. The incidence is approximately one case per year per million of population. Commonly beginning as an ascending paralysis, it is often associated with paraesthesia and may progress to involve the respiratory (30%) and bulbar muscles (8%). Respiratory muscle involvement leads to a fall in lung volumes, especially VC. Commonly, false reassurance is gained by measuring either blood gases, which may be normal until late in the disease process, or forced expiratory volume in 1 s (FEV_1), a parameter that does not predict ventilatory capacity.

Autonomic nervous system involvement often leads to dysrhythmias, labile blood pressure, ileus, urinary retention and abnormal thermoregulation. In the Miller–Fischer variant, there is a triad of ataxia, areflexia and ophthalmoplegia, but crossover between this and the more 'typical' presentation is well recognised. Other cranial nerves, especially the seventh, may be affected.

The pathophysiology of Guillain–Barré syndrome remains unclear, but an auto-immune response to Schwann cells or peripheral nerve myelin is thought to occur. In the early phase of the illness, neurophysiological testing may be inconclusive, but as it progresses, patchy demyelination and axonal degeneration become apparent. Nerve conduction velocity is reduced (Figure 15.1).

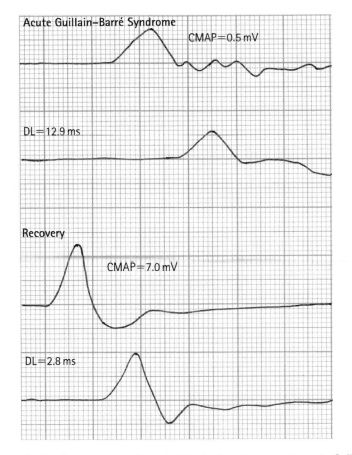

Figure 15.1 – Reduced nerve conduction velocities in the ulnar nerve in acute Guillain–Barré syndrome and following recovery. Note the prolongation of the distal latency (DL, normal value <3 ms), reduction and prolongation of the compound muscle action potential (CMAP, normal value >5 mV in the ulnar nerve).

In a patient with a typical history, a raised cerebrospinal fluid protein (>3 g.l⁻¹) is strongly suggestive of the diagnosis, but this may take up to a week to develop, and false negative results may be obtained if the lumbar puncture is performed early.

Other diagnoses that should be considered include motor neurone disease, myasthenia gravis, Eaton–Lambert syndrome, diphtheria, poliomyelitis, botulism and severe inorganic lead poisoning (Table 15.1).

Motor neurone disease is usually of more insidious onset, and is associated with widespread muscle fasciculation. Myasthenia gravis is usually associated with other autoimmune conditions and characteristically causes ptosis and generalised muscle weakness without paraesthesia. The administration of a short acting anticholinergic

Table 15.1 – Differential diagnosis of acute neuromuscular failure.

Condition	Cause	Site affected	Sensory versus motor	Autonomic dysfunction	Diagnosis	Treatment
Guillain–Barré syndrome	Viral or bacterial infection Immunisation Surgery	Peripheral nerves	M > S	Common	CSF protein rise Electrodiagnostic	Supportive care Intravenous gamma-globulin Plasmapheresis
Myasthenia Gravis	Autoimmune	Neuromuscular junction	M	Absent	Anticholinesterase test	Anticholinesterase therapy Thymectomy Immunosuppression
Eaton–Lambert syndrome	Underlying malignancy Antibody to presynaptic calcium receptor	Neuromuscular junction	M	Common	Associated autonomic dysfunction Electrodiagnostic	Treat underlying cause Immunosuppression Plasmapheresis
Poliomyelitis	Poliovirus	Anterior horn cells	S > M	Common	CSF pleocytosis Stool culture Electrodiagnostic	Supportive care
Motor neurone disease	Unknown	Motor neurones	M	Absent	Clinical	None
Botulism	Botulinum toxin	Binding to receptors on unmyelinated pre-synaptic membrane	M	Common	Electrodiagnostic (incremental response to stimulation)	Antitoxin Wound debridement Penicillin
Diphtheria	Corynebacterium diphtheriae	Peripheral nerves	S > M	Parasympathetic depression	Culture from throat or skin ulcer	Antitoxin
Inorganic lead poisoning	Lead ingestion	Motor or sensory peripheral nerves	M > S	Absent	Lead levels Electrodiagnostic	Remove source Chelating agents

agents (e.g. edrophomium 2 mg intravenously, followed by up to 8 mg) will often produce a dramatic improvement in muscle strength, thereby confirming the diagnosis of myasthenia. The Eaton–Lambert syndrome is similar to myasthenia gravis, but is associated with malignancy (e.g. carcinoma of the lung); however, weakness does not improve after the administration of anticholinergic drugs. Diphtheria can usually be differentiated on the basis of the severe sore throat and associated systemic illness. Botulism arises from the ingestion of botulinum toxin and is usually characterised by an acute gastrointestinal disturbance associated with rapidly progressive generalised paralysis. Poliomyelitis is rare in immunised adults, but transmission of live virus between recently immunised infants and non-immunised adults can occur. Poliomyelitis is associated with asymmetrical paralysis, usually accompanied by muscle pain and a systemic febrile illness. Organic lead poisoning is rare and is usually associated with some form of occupational exposure.

THERAPEUTIC GOALS

The therapeutic goals in this patient are:

1. It is essential that the airway is secured to prevent aspiration and respiratory tract soiling. Hypoxaemia and hypercapnia should be corrected using oxygen therapy and intermittent positive pressure ventilation.

2. The circulation should be optimised using intravenous fluids and vaso-active drugs. Autonomic disturbances affecting the heart rate and blood pressure may require treatment.

3. Provision of adequate analgesia, sedation and anxiolysis is essential.

4. Infection should be treated with antibiotics. Regular pulmonary and limb physiotherapy is essential.

5. Thorough consideration of the differential diagnosis is essential.

6. Attention must be given to nutrition, the care of skin and joints, body temperature and the psychological welfare of the patient.

7. Specific therapies (e.g. plasmapheresis or intravenous gamma-globulin therapy) should be commenced.

THERAPEUTIC OPTIONS BASED ON PHYSIOLOGICAL AND PHARMACOLOGICAL EFFECTS

In the emergency phase, stabilisation of the patient's airway, breathing and circulation takes precedence over any investigations.

Airway

Emergency intubation and ventilation may be especially hazardous in a patient with hypoxaemia, hypercapnia and hypotension. In patients with autonomic dysfunction, the risk is increased by dysrhythmias, blood pressure lability and gastric paresis (i.e. increased danger of regurgitation and aspiration of gastric residue).

While preparing equipment and drugs, the blood pressure should be restored by fluid challenges and/or the commencing of inotropic support (e.g. dobutamine $5–10\,\mu\text{g.kg.min}^{-1}$). The administration of a positively chronotropic agent will reduce the risk of autonomic bradycardia during airway manipulation.

A rapid sequence intubation should be performed after pre-oxygenation. All induction agents, except ketamine and etomidate, are liable to cause hypotension. However, with careful titration of induction agent, intravenous fluid boluses and inotropic support, significant hypotension can usually be avoided. Suxamethonium should not be used to facilitate intubation, because potassium release from denervated muscles may produce life threatening hyperkalaemia. A 'modified' rapid sequence intubation using rocuronium ($1\,\text{mg.kg}^{-1}$) in combination with alfentanil ($10–15\,\mu\text{g.kg}^{-1}$) will rapidly produce good intubating conditions.

Awake fibre-optic intubation under local anaesthesia may be appropriate if the patient is cooperative, the coagulation screen is normal and the operator is experienced in the technique. The naso-tracheal route tends to be easier and is better tolerated by the patient. The technique can be performed with the patient sitting upright, thereby reducing the risk of regurgitation and aspiration of gastric contents.

Tracheostomy is sensibly deferred until there is some indication of the likely time course of the disease process. Some patients respond rapidly to specific treatment and the need for tracheostomy may therefore be avoided. However, if there is clinical evidence of bulbar dysfunction, a tracheostomy may be necessary early on, irrespective of the ventilatory reserve.

Breathing

Patients with Guillain–Barré syndrome managed on general hospital wards should be closely observed for respiratory distress, and monitoring of VC is mandatory. Blood gas abnormalities are a late sign of the need for ventilatory support. VC should be measured hourly; a deteriorating trend in VC or a single value of less than 1 l is an indication for mechanical ventilation.

In practice, many patients will have a degree of atelectasis and it is common for high levels of positive end expiratory pressure (PEEP) to be required for lung recruitment measures during the first few hours of mechanical ventilation. Careful titration of analgesia and anxiolysis may allow patients to be managed either awake or minimally sedated as the depressed bulbar reflexes makes the patient more tolerant of the tracheal tube.

In some circumstances, if the bulbar reflexes are intact there may be a role for non-invasive ventilatory support using a nasal mask or close fitting face mask. Many patients have a limited ability to tolerate such devices, particularly, if they have asso-ciated confusion or agitation. However, the dangers of aspiration remain high.

Circulation

Different causes of circulatory instability may co-exist in patients with Guillain–Barré syndrome. Those who have been unwell for several days may have had a reduced oral intake and may be dehydrated. Associated diarrhoea and vomiting, due to autonomic dysfunction, may exacerbate hypovolaemia. Pulmonary sepsis and the associated inflammatory response may cause venodilation with sequestration of cir-culating fluids; circulating cytokines may depress myocardial contractility. Auto-nomic dysfunction also causes vasoparesis and may lead to bradycardia and heart block. Less commonly, it causes hypertensive crises and tachyarrhythmias.

The patient will require restoration of circulating volume, and possibly, vasoactive drugs to optimise cardiac, cerebral, renal and splanchnic perfusion. Central venous access is usually essential, and it may be helpful to monitor cardiac output during the initial phases of the disease. Specific therapy for symptomatic bradycardia may include anticholinergic agents such as atropine (0.20 $\mu g.kg^{-1}$) or glycopyrrolate ($20–40$ $\mu g.kg^{-1}$). Heart block is rare, but may respond to infusion of isoprenaline ($0.1–2$ $\mu g.kg^{-1}.min^{-1}$) or require temporary pacing.

It is important to identify autonomic dysfunction as there are many common causes of dysrhythmias and blood pressure variation. Other causes include inade-quate sedation or analgesia, excessive inotropic support and inadequate ventilation (carbon dioxide retention is a potent stimulant of catecholamine secretion). If more obvious causes have been excluded, it may be necessary to give nifedip-ine ($5–20$ mg, sublingual or oral), glycerine trinitrate ($1–10$ $\mu g.kg^{-1}.min^{-1}$) or angiotensinogen converting enzyme inhibitors for hypertension, and β-blockers such as propranolol for tachycardia. Labetalol ($0.2–2$ $mg.kg^{-1}.h^{-1}$) may be particu-larly advantageous if hypertension and tachycardia co-exist, as it produces com-bined α-adrenergic and β-adrenergic receptor blockade.

Analgesia sedation and anxiolysis

In deciding which sedative agents to use, the likely time course of the patient's intensive care management should be considered. There may be benefits in choos-ing short acting agents if a short duration of respiratory support is anticipated. If it is clear that a long stay and early tracheostomy are likely, long acting sedatives are preferable. Muscle relaxants should be avoided other than for procedures such as intubation, and great care should be taken to ensure that all carers are aware of the risks associated with the use of suxamethonium in such patients. During plasma exchange, sedative drugs may be cleared rapidly and may cause unwanted emer-gence from sedation.

Muscle and joint pain is a common feature of Guillain–Barré syndrome and should be treated sympathetically. Simple analgesics (e.g. paracetamol (15–20 mg.kg^{-1} orally or rectally)) should be used initially, but stronger analgesics such as non-steroidal anti-inflammatory agents, tramadol (50–100 mg orally or intravenously) or even opioids may occasionally be required.

Pulmonary infection

The most important aspect of care is the prevention of pulmonary soiling by early protection of the airway. If aspiration of pharyngeal or gastric contents is suspected, the initial therapy includes airway protection, ventilatory support and microbiological surveillance. Sputum clearance and physiotherapy probably have more to offer than antibiotics at this stage. If there is clinical evidence of pulmonary infection, identification of the causal organism should be attempted prior to the administration of antibiotics. Non-bronchoscopic lavage (NBL) is generally the most reliable means of isolating pulmonary pathogens. The decision to treat depends on the patient's condition, the presence or absence of infected sputum, the identification of new areas of bronchial breathing in non-dependant areas of lung, pyrexia or elevated c-reactive protein levels, or a raised white cell count. The choice of antibiotic regimen should take into account local microbiological epidemiology and resistance patterns.

Nutritional support

Having been unwell for at least a week, during which he will have been unable to eat, this patient will require nutritional support. Patients with Guillain–Barré syndrome who require ventilation will usually absorb enteral feed administered through a naso-gastric tube. For comfort a fine-bore tube should be inserted in patients who are being managed with little or no sedation. Care should be taken in confirming the correct position of the tip of the tube as translaryngeal passage is possible even with a tracheal tube in place. However, sometimes, autonomic dysfunction prevents absorption of enteral feed; if so, a naso-jejunal tube may help, although parenteral nutrition may be required. In patients with a protracted clinical course, an endoscopically-assisted percutaneous gastrostomy tube may ultimately be necessary.

Deep vein thrombosis prophylaxis

There is good clinical evidence that the incidence of thromboembolic complications is reduced by prophylactic measures, and their use reduces the risk of death for patients with Guillain–Barré syndrome. Regular physiotherapy and mobilisation are important; compression stockings may also be useful. However, heparin prophylaxis is essential. Low-molecular weight heparin prophylaxis may be preferable in terms of patient comfort as it reduces the frequency of subcutaneous injection.

Specific therapies

Intravenous gamma-globulin therapy (IVIG) $(0.4\,\mathrm{g.kg}^{-1}.\mathrm{day}^{-1}$ for between 3 and 6 days) has been shown to effectively reduce the rate of deterioration in Guillain–Barré syndrome and in hastening neurological recovery. There appears to be a 'therapeutic window' of approximately 2 weeks from the onset of symptoms, during which the benefits of intravenous gamma-globulin therapy may be greatest. Intravenous gamma-globulin therapy is derived from blood products and therefore carries theoretical risks of disease transmission. Anaphylactic reactions are recognised but rare.

Plasma exchange has also been shown to reduce the duration of symptoms and to speed recovery in Guillain–Barré syndrome. There appears to be a similar treatment 'window' as for intravenous gamma-globulin therapy. There is no clear data to guide the volume of plasma exchange undertaken, its frequency or the total number of treatments that are necessary. A pragmatic approach is to perform two plasma-volume exchanges on five consecutive days. There is some evidence that a second course of plasma exchange may be of benefit if the clinical condition subsequently relapses. Plasma exchange can readily be performed in most intensive care units by using a plasma filter in a pumped circuit similar to that used for continuous veno-venous haemofiltration. The major complication is hypotension as a consequence of failure to match the rate of plasma removal with volume replacement, but the general risks of any extra-corporeal circulation exist (e.g. haemorrhage from the venous access site, air embolism) are also present as well. No clear evidence exists of the superiority of either intravenous gamma-globulin therapy or plasma exchange. Consequently, the relative simplicity of intravenous gamma-globulin therapy means that it should probably be tried before plasma exchange.

There is considerable interest in the technique of cerebrospinal fluid filtration in Guillain–Barré syndrome, and some evidence that it may be of benefit in patients with chronic manifestations of the disease. A European trial of cerebrospinal fluid filtration in acute Guillain–Barré syndrome is currently in progress. The theoretical basis is that cerebrospinal fluid of Guillain–Barré syndrome sufferers contains a sodium-channel blocking agent which can be removed by filtration.

USUAL OUTCOME

The severity and time course of Guillain–Barré syndrome is very variable. There is evidence that patients with a more rapid onset of paralysis are more likely to have a prolonged disease course and are more likely to have an incomplete recovery. Some patients will avoid the need for airway protection or mechanical ventilation, and many of those who require it will respond within days to specific therapy. Less fortunate patients may require treatment extending to weeks or even months, and a small percentage may remain severely disabled. Longer duration is associated with advancing age and with a gastrointestinal prodromal illness, particularly if caused by *Campylobacter*. Outcome is improved by high quality nursing care, attention to detail, and avoidance of complications. The detection of severe axonal degeneration (as opposed to demyelination) suggests a particularly prolonged duration of paralysis and that recovery is unlikely to be complete.

The prognosis for recovery from Guillain–Barré syndrome is generally good, and 85% of patients make a complete or near complete recovery. The majority of the remainder may have mild residual neurological weakness or paraesthesiae. The mortality is 3–4%. Less than 1% of patients may fail to improve despite specific therapy and progress to chronic inflammatory demyelinating polyneuropathy, which may have devastating implications for their long-term health, including permanent ventilator dependence, paraplegia and quadriplegia.

KEY LEARNING POINTS

1. Patients with Guillain–Barré syndrome are vulnerable to sudden respiratory decompensation if bulbar muscles are involved.

2. VC is a better indicator of severity than blood gas analyses or FEV_1.

3. Suxamethonium should be avoided as it may produce severe hyperkalaemia.

4. Intravenous immunoglobulin and plasmapheresis are both effective treatments.

5. The mortality rate should be low if patients receive early intervention and high quality supportive care.

Further reading

1. Hughes RAC. The Guillain Barré syndrome. *Prescribers' Journal* 1998; **38**: 167–74.

2. Krull F, Schudhardt V, Haupt WF, Mewes J. Prognosis of acute polyneuritis requiring artificial ventilation. *Intensive Care Medicine* 1988; **14**: 388–92.

3. Ropper AH. The Guillain Barré syndrome. *New England Journal of Medicine* 1992; **326**: 1130–6.

4. Rantala H, Uhari M, Niemela M. Occurrence, clinical manifestations and prognosis of Guillain Barré syndrome. *Archives of Disease in Childhood* 1991; **66**: 706–9.

5. Guillain Barré Study Group. Plasmapheresis and acute GBS. *Neurology* 1985; **35**: 1096–104.

6. Alter M. The epidemiology of Guillain Barré syndrome. *Annals of Neurology* 1990; **27**: S7–S12.

7. Wollinsky KH, Hulser PJ, Brinkmeier H *et al.* CSF filtration is an effective treatment of Guillain Barré syndrome; a randomised clinical trial. *Neurology* 2001; **57**: 774–80.

8. Brinkmeir H, Wollinsky KH, Hulser PJ *et al.* The acute paralysis in Guillain Barré syndrome is related to a Na$^+$ channel blocking factor in the cerebrospinal fluid. *European Journal of Physiology* 1992; **421**: 552–7.

9. El-shunnar K. Guillain Barre syndrome: a neurosurgical experience. *British Medical Journal* **302**: 1473–4.

10. Hughes RAC, Bihari D. Acute neuromuscular respiratory paralysis. In: Hughes RAC (ed.), *Neurological emergencies,* 2nd edn. London: BMJ Publishing, 1997: 295–319.

16

A 19-YEAR-OLD FEMALE WITH ACUTE SEVERE ASTHMA

P Phipps & C S Garrard

CASE SCENARIO

A 19-year-old asthmatic female presents to the Accident and Emergency (A&E) Department with a 2-day history of increasing cough, wheeze and dyspnoea. Her usual medications of salbutamol and fluticasone inhaler have been ineffective and she has worsened despite receiving nebulised salbutamol and 50 mg prednisolone from her general practitioner this morning. She does not smoke and is otherwise well. Her asthma is usually well controlled with regular high dose inhaled corticosteroids and salbutamol as required; her general practitioner says she is compliant with her medication. She has required four courses of oral corticosteroids in the past year. Her last hospital admission was 3 months ago. However, 8 months ago, she was admitted to the intensive care unit (ICU) with a severe exacerbation that required 2 days of mechanical ventilation.

In the A&E Department, she continues to deteriorate, despite nebulised salbutamol (5 mg hourly) and ipratropium (500 µg), and intravenous hydrocortisone (200 mg). She is tachypnoeic, distressed and is only able to speak in single words. She was hypoxaemic on room air with a saturation of 90%, which increased with oxygen.

DEFINITION AND DESCRIPTION OF THE PROBLEM

Asthma is reversible airflow obstruction due to airway inflammation that typically presents with exacerbations, the majority of which can be managed in the Community or Emergency Department. More severe cases (i.e. those that do not respond to initial therapy) require admission to a high dependency unit (HDU) or ICU. Overall, hospital and ICU admission rates are increasing, but mortality rates are falling. Prompt and careful assessment, close monitoring and appropriate therapy are required to minimise morbidity and mortality.

Risk factors for mortality and assessment of severity

A history of near-fatal asthma and mechanical ventilation are markers for subsequent asthma death. Patients who present late, and those who deteriorate despite optimal treatment, are at particular risk. Other general risk factors for a life threatening episode include female gender (adult females are more susceptible to both life threatening attacks and asthma deaths), low socio-economic status, psychosocial factors and smoking history (Table 16.1).

Table 16.1 – Risk factors for asthma morbidity and mortality.

Prior history of near-fatal asthma
Deterioration despite oral corticosteroids
Older age (>55 years)
Co-morbidity (e.g. heart disease)
Smokers
Low socio-economic status
Isolation from medical care
Psychosocial problems

Worrying examination findings include impaired conscious level, inability to speak, use of accessory muscles and diaphoresis. Similarly, the degree of tachypnoea, tachycardia and pulsus paradoxus gives an indication of the severity of the attack. Tracheal deviation, asymmetric breath sounds or subcutaneous emphysema suggest a pneumothorax, which should be treated promptly.

Although signs of respiratory distress will be evident in the early phases of acute severe asthma, patients may become drowsy and look more comfortable as the condition worsens; also accessory muscle use, wheeze, pulsus paradoxus and tachypnoea may diminish. Objective measures of severity include spirometry, oximetry, arterial blood-gas analysis, chest radiography and electrocardiogram (ECG). Careful and regular clinical assessment is essential. The criteria for immediate intubation are cardiopulmonary arrest, near-cardiopulmonary arrest (i.e. being unable to speak, gasping for air), coma or a significantly obtunded mental state. Other causes of respiratory distress, such as left ventricular failure, upper airway obstruction, inhaled foreign body and aspiration of stomach contents should be excluded.

PATHOLOGY AND PATHOPHYSIOLOGY OF ACUTE SEVERE ASTHMA

Post-mortem studies of patients dying of acute severe asthma demonstrate extensive mucus plugging of bronchi; this is termed endobronchial mucus suffocation.

Microscopy reveals extensive inflammatory changes involving all airway wall components and the pulmonary arterioles. Mucus, desquamated epithelium, inflammatory cells and plasma exudate contribute to bronchial occlusion. In contrast, sudden asphyxic asthma is thought to be a distinct pathological subtype in which intense bronchoconstriction causes respiratory failure, often over the course of 1–2 h. Recovery appears to be rapid suggesting that bronchoconstriction may be the predominant pathophysiological factor.

Expiratory airflow limitation produces a dynamic increase in end-expiratory lung volume, which interferes with inspiratory muscle function. The positive alveolar pressure at end expiration due to residual elastic recoil has been termed intrinsic positive end-expiratory pressure ($PEEP_i$). Its presence is suggested by residual expiratory flow at the onset of inspiration (Figure 16.1).

Many patients also use expiratory muscles to aid expiration, which may paradoxically worsen dynamic airway collapse and $PEEP_i$. The pathological effects of airflow limitation and $PEEP_i$ include ventilation : perfusion inequality, respiratory muscle fatigue due to the high work of breathing, reduced venous return and an increased risk of pneumothorax. These lead to hypoxaemia, hypercapnia and hypotension.

THERAPEUTIC GOALS

The therapeutic goals in a patient with severe asthma include:

1. Reversal of bronchoconstriction.

2. Relief of airway inflammation.

3. Avoidance of complications such as hypoxaemia, electrolyte abnormalities, dehydration, pneumothorax and arrhythmias.

The presence of severe airflow limitation (peak expiratory flow rate (PEFR) <33% predicted or forced expiratory volume in 1 s (FEV_1) <1 l), signs of fatigue (i.e. rising P_aCO_2, difficulty speaking, altered mental state), cardiovascular instability or a requirement for intravenous bronchodilators necessitates intensive monitoring on the HDU or ICU.

THERAPEUTIC OPTIONS BASED ON PHYSIOLOGICAL AND PHARMACODYNAMIC EFFECTS

Patients who fail to improve rapidly with optimal medical therapy in the A&E Department should be considered for HDU or ICU admission, especially if there is, as in this case, a previous history of ICU admission. HDU or ICU admission greatly facilitates continuous monitoring of the patient's clinical condition and

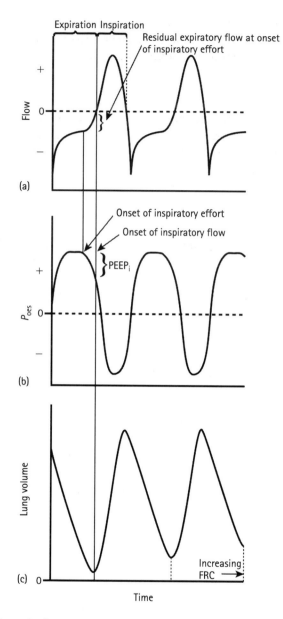

Figure 16.1 – Schematic diagram of an asthmatic patient exhibiting significant residual flow at end expiration (a). The oesophageal pressure, an estimate of intrapleural pressure, demonstrates the degree of pressure change required to overcome $PEEP_i$ and initiate inspiratory flow (b). A progressive increase in lung volume (breath stacking) occurs, if expiratory time is insufficient to allow complete exhalation of the tidal volume (c). (Reproduced with permission from Rossi A, Ganassini A, Polese G, Grassi V. Pulmonary hyperinflation and ventilator dependent patients. *European Respiratory Journal* 1997; **10**: 1663–74.)

physiological parameters such as pulse oximetry, ECG and arterial and central venous pressure. Equipment and experienced staff are also readily available for procedures such as tracheal intubation or tube thoracocentesis.

Initial therapy

Adequate oxygenation is paramount; a high concentration of inhaled oxygen (via a non-re-breathing face mask) should be supplied to asthmatics to keep oxygen saturation above 95%. This is in contrast to patients with chronic obstructive lung disease, who may be dependent on a hypoxaemic respiratory drive where oxygen therapy may need to be more limited.

Corticosteroids and β-adrenergic receptor agonists are first line therapy. An initial intravenous dose of hydrocortisone (200 mg) followed by 100 mg every 6 h or 50 mg of oral prednisolone daily should be commenced immediately. Higher doses do not confer additional benefit and the intravenous route should be used if the patient is unable to tolerate or is unlikely to absorb an oral dose. Inhaled corticosteroids have not been fully evaluated in the severe asthmatic admitted to intensive care.

β-Adrenergic receptor agonists are the most effective when inhaled and, therefore, continuous administration of nebulised salbutamol in doses approaching $20 \, \text{mg.h}^{-1}$ should be used. Continuous ECG monitoring is essential, although cardio-toxicity from this regimen is unusual and the heart rate may even fall with clinical improvement. Although bronchodilators delivered by metred dose inhaler with a spacer device are at least as effective as nebulised drugs in the management of acute asthma, nebulised drugs may be easier to administer in patients with hypoxaemia and respiratory distress. Long-acting β-adrenergic receptor agonists are not recommended because of their slow onset of action. Ipratropium bromide has a mild additional bronchodilating effect when added to β-adrenergic receptor agonists in severe asthma, so a 500 μg dose every 2–4 h should be commenced.

Second line agents

There are a number of second line agents that can be used. Nebulised and intravenous adrenaline (epinephrine) are effective in acute asthma therapy, although there does not appear to be any proven clinical benefit over selective β-adrenergic receptor agonists, such as salbutamol. Early parenteral adrenaline is, however, indicated in cases of anaphylaxis.

If there is no improvement after using the above regimen, an intravenous bronchodilator (aminophylline or salbutamol) should be added, although there is some doubt as to the benefit. Side effects and complication rates of these intravenous drugs are significant.

Other bronchodilator agents

There have been inconsistent reports of benefit from intravenous magnesium sulphate in doses of 1 or 2 g in acute severe asthma and it is currently not recommended in the British Thoracic Society Guidelines. Hypomagneseamia should, however, be treated to reduce the risk of arrhythmias.

Leucotriene antagonists such as montelukast (10 mg, orally or 7 mg, intravenously) improve lung function and may reduce the need for hospital or ICU admission of asthmatics.

Assisted ventilation

If there is inadequate response to asthma therapy, improving gas exchange using assisted ventilation may be life saving.

In spontaneously breathing asthmatics, continuous positive airways pressure (CPAP) at low levels (3–8 cmH$_2$O) delivered by face mask may improve respiratory rate, dyspnoea and the work of breathing. Non-invasive ventilation, providing both positive inspiratory pressure support and CPAP, may improve gas exchange and avoid intubation in hypercapnic asthmatics. However, there is a risk that lung hyperinflation may worsen. If the patient is deteriorating rapidly or has an altered conscious state, intubation should not be delayed.

Intubation

Understanding of the pathophysiology and anticipating difficulties can minimise the complications associated with tracheal intubation and ventilation. The process of intubation begins with explanation and re-assurance for the patient, followed by pre-oxygenation. The asthmatic patient may often be dehydrated and the combination of hyperinflation, the loss of endogenous catecholamines and the vasodilating properties of the sedative agents can cause a catastrophic, and potentially fatal, fall in blood pressure. Volume resuscitation and correction of electrolyte abnormalities prior to induction of anaesthesia can limit the degree of hypotension and arrhythmias. Occasionally, vasoconstrictors such as ephedrine or metaraminol may be required temporarily and should be readily available.

Intubation is best performed by direct laryngoscopy after rapid sequence induction of general anaesthesia. Endoscopic methods have been advocated, but laryngeal spasm and further bronchoconstriction may occur even in the presence of adequate local anaesthesia of the oropharynx and larynx. Longer term sedation will be required once the airway has been secured.

A range of agents, including etomidate and thiopentone, can be safely used for the induction of anaesthesia prior to intubation, although rare bronchospasm and anaphylactoid reactions have been reported. Other useful agents for the induction of anaesthesia, and subsequent sedation include propofol, midazolam and ketamine.

Ketamine has both sympathomimetic and bronchodilating properties, but it may increase blood pressure and heart rate, lower seizure threshold and cause delirium. Inhalational anaesthetics for gaseous induction have the advantage of bronchodilation and may make muscle relaxation unnecessary. However, familiarity with the technique and specialised anaesthetic equipment is required.

Opioids are a useful adjunct to sedatives as they can provide analgesia during intubation and mechanical ventilation. However, morphine causes histamine release in large doses, which may worsen bronchoconstriction and hypotension. Some intravenous morphine preparations also contain metabisulphite, to which some asthmatics are sensitive. Fentanyl is a better choice of opioid as it inhibits airway reflexes, is short acting and causes much less histamine release than morphine. However, in large doses it may cause bronchospasm and chest wall rigidity.

Muscle relaxation will usually be required during intubation and the depolarising agent, suxamethonium ($1-2\,\text{mg.kg}^{-1}$) is widely used. It has a rapid onset and short duration of action, but may cause hyperkalaemia and increased intracranial pressure. Rocuronium, a non-depolarising muscle relaxant with a rapid onset offers an alternative. Allergic sensitivity may occur to any neuromuscular blocking agent and most may also cause histamine release, risking bronchospasm, particularly in bolus doses. Atracurium boluses should be avoided because of this possibility. Longer term maintenance of muscle relaxation after intubation can be achieved with an infusion of vecuronium or intermittent doses of pancuronium. It should be noted that myopathy and muscle weakness have been extensively reported following medium- to long-term administration of non-depolarising neuromuscular blocking agents in asthmatics. The incidence is approximately 30%, so the use of neuromuscular blocking agents should be kept to a minimum. Recommendations for intubation are summarised in Table 16.2.

Table 16.2 – Summary of recommendations for the process of intubation.

Performed/supervised by experienced anaesthetists/intensivists
Skilled assistants in an appropriate environment
Good preparation and understanding of the pathophysiology
Correct electrolyte disturbances and rehydration
Reliable large bore venous access
Continuous ECG and pulse oximetry
Continuous arterial monitoring not essential, but helpful
Pre-oxygenation
Use familiar method of intubation
Use familiar sedatives and muscle relaxants
Prepare for the rapid correction of hypotension, arrhythmias and barotrauma
Set up ventilator and be ready to monitor airway pressures early
Prepare aerosol delivery system for the ventilator or commence parenteral bronchodilator
Plan ongoing sedation/paralysis prior to intubation

Ventilator settings

Commonly adopted ventilation modes include pressure-limited (pressure control or bilevel ventilation) or volume-limited modes (synchronised intermittent mandatory ventilation). In pressure-limited modes, target inspiratory pressures are set and the tidal volume delivered depends on respiratory system compliance. Volume-limited modes, however, deliver a set tidal volume and the airway pressure generated may be high. Volume-limited modes may be safely used, provided an airway pressure limit is set appropriately. As the patient improves and begins to breathe, spontaneously triggered modes of ventilation, such as pressure support ventilation can be introduced.

Outcome is improved in mechanically ventilated asthmatics by limiting airway pressures using a low respiratory rate and tidal volume, while permitting a small to moderate degree of hypercapnia. Reducing the respiratory rate to 8 or 10 breaths.min^{-1} prolongs expiratory time so that inspiratory to expiratory (I:E) ratios of greater than 1:2 can be achieved. Humidification of inspired gas is particularly important in asthmatic patients, to prevent thickening of secretions and drying of airway mucosa, which is a stimulus for bronchospasm itself. Initial ventilator settings are suggested in Table 16.3.

Table 16.3 – Recommended initial ventilator settings in paralysed or heavily sedated patients.

$F_iO_2 = 1$ (initially)
Long expiratory time (I:E ratio 1:2 to 1:4)
Low tidal volume 5–7 ml.kg^{-1}
Low ventilator rate 10 cycles.min^{-1}
Set inspiratory pressure 30–35 cmH_2O on pressure control ventilation or limit peak inspiratory pressure <40 cmH_2O
Minimal or no PEEP

Ventilator alarm settings such as peak pressure and low tidal volume should be carefully selected. If exceptionally high airway pressures occur, or there is a sudden fall in tidal volume, blockage of the tracheal tube, pneumothorax or lobar collapse may be the cause.

Low level CPAP may be beneficial in spontaneously breathing, mechanically assisted patients, especially if expiratory muscle activity is contributing to dynamic airways collapse. However, in mechanically ventilated, paralysed patients, externally applied PEEP is of no benefit at low levels and detrimental at high levels because the fall in gas trapping is outweighed by a rise in functional residual capacity.

Bronchodilator administration in ventilated patients

Once mechanical ventilation has commenced, the delivery of aerosolised bronchodilator may be seriously impaired. The amount of drug reaching the patients'

Table 16.4 – Recommendations for aerosol delivery to mechanically ventilated patients.

(a) Metred dose inhaler (MDI) system
Spacer or holding chamber
Location in inspiratory limb rather than Y piece
No humidification (briefly discontinue)
Activate during lung inflation
Large tracheal tube internal diameter
Prolonged inspiratory time
(b) Jet-nebuliser system
Mount nebuliser in inspiratory limb
Delivery may be improved by inspiratory triggering
Increase inspiratory time and decrease respiratory rate
Use a spacer
High flow to generate aerosol
High volume fill
Stop humidification
Consider continuous nebulisation
(c) Ultrasonic nebulisers
Position in inspiratory limb prior to a spacer device
Use high power setting
Use a high volume fill
Maximise inspiratory time
Drugs must be stable during ultrasonic nebulisation

airways depends on the nebuliser design, driving gas flow, configuration of the ventilator tubing, the presence of humidification and the size of the tracheal tube. The dose should therefore be increased to ensure a therapeutic benefit or until side effects become apparent. Some ultrasonic nebulisers work well in ventilated patients, but can be the source of bacterial contamination. Recommendations for inhalation therapy in intubated patients are provided in Table 16.4.

Metered dose inhalers have been widely used and may provide at least as good drug delivery as nebulisers, depending on actuator design and the presence of humidification and spacer devices. Each aerosol delivery system needs to be evaluated for efficiency in each type of ventilator circuit used.

Strategies in non-responding patients

If patients deteriorate or do not improve, ineffective drug delivery or complications such as pneumothorax should be considered. If the deterioration is acute with hypotension, desaturation, low tidal volumes and subcutaneous emphysema, a chest drain should be urgently placed without waiting for a confirmatory chest X-ray. If there is any doubt about lateralising signs, bilateral chest drains should be inserted. If the deterioration is rapid, unilateral or bilateral needles or cannulae can be placed in the second intercostal space, mid-clavicular line and chest drains inserted immediately thereafter. If a bronchopleural fistula occurs, the ventilator can compensate for the loss in tidal volume. Closure of the fistula often does not begin until the patient has been weaned from mechanical ventilation.

Difficulty in ventilation is usually due to refractory bronchospasm, extreme hyper-inflation or mucus plugging. As other ventilator settings can lead to air trapping and difficulties with ventilation, a low tidal volume, low respiratory rate and an I : E ratio of >1 : 2 should be applied.

The relief of intense hyperinflation may be achieved by manual compression of the chest wall during expiration. The technique has been advocated and used with success in both intubated and non-intubated patients, although it has not been fully evaluated.

Mucus impaction in the airways often contributes to hyperinflation, segmental and lobar collapse and barotrauma. Chest physiotherapy and mucolytics have no proven benefit, but bronchoscopic lavage using n-acetylcysteine may clear impacted secretions in patients exhibiting X-ray evidence of segmental collapse or sputum containing mucus plugs (unrelieved by chest physiotherapy) and bronchoscopic evidence of mucus impaction.

A number of volatile anaesthetic agents such as halothane, isoflurane and sevoflu-rane are potent bronchodilators in asthmatics receiving mechanical ventilation. They rapidly reduce peak airway pressures, improve ventilation distribution and reduce air trapping. These agents also offer a convenient, although relatively expen-sive, method of sedation. Side effects such as hypotension and myocardial irritabil-ity can occur. The Seimens Servo 900 ventilator can be fitted with a vaporiser and an exhaled gas scavenging system so that volatile agents can be conveniently admin-istered in the ICU.

Other agents that have been used include helium and oxygen mixtures (Heliox) and nitric oxide. Heliox may reduce the work of breathing and improve gas exchange due to its low density, but the benefits are marginal and may com-promise the amount of inspired oxygen that can be delivered. Nitric oxide exerts a weak bronchodilator effect and dilates pulmonary arteries; when inhaled, it may improve ventilation : perfusion matching and oxygenation.

Weaning and extubation

One of the difficult aspects of mechanical ventilation of the acute asthmatic is the weaning and extubation process. The presence of the tracheal tube induces bron-choconstriction, which becomes troublesome as the sedation is withdrawn in the preparation for extubation. By using an inhalation anaesthetic agent, the tracheal tube can be removed under anaesthesia with the confident expectation of rapid recovery, once the anaesthetic is discontinued.

USUAL OUTCOME

In the initial stages of an attack, difficulty in establishing a secure airway, baro-trauma, arrhythmias and ventilator associated infection may all lead to morbidity and mortality in asthmatics. Sadly, respiratory arrest leading to hypoxic brain injury continues to occur in asthma, either in the pre-hospital setting, or if in-hospital monitoring and treatment is inadequate.

Although deaths from asthma in hospital are fortunately rare, an ICU admission identifies an asthmatic as a member of a poor prognostic group. Post intensive care mortality has been reported at 10% at 1 year and 23% after 6 years. The patient should, therefore, be managed for a suitable period by both intensive care and medical teams prior to and after discharge from ICU. The respiratory team prior to hospital discharge will provide intense anti-inflammatory therapy and a management plan that may include the emergency use of intramuscular adrenaline. Close medical follow-up will be arranged and issues such as access to health care services, compliance with therapy, allergens or triggers in the home environment, socio-economic and psychosocial factors will all need to be addressed.

KEY LEARNING POINTS

1. Ensure early recognition of poor prognostic factors from history and physical examination.

2. Optimise therapy early by including high oxygen concentration, continuously nebulised bronchodilators, steroids and intravenous bronchodilators. Review response to therapy regularly.

3. Consider early transfer to HDU or ICU for close monitoring of physiological parameters and early detection of complications.

4. Involve an experienced clinician to intubate with prior oxygenation, hydration and correction of electrolyte abnormalities.

5. Use a ventilation strategy to minimise complications and improve outcome (i.e. low tidal volume and long expiratory time while accepting moderate hypercarbia).

6. Consider other therapies such as inhaled anaesthetics, manual chest compression or bronchoscopy.

7. Follow-up requires specialist respiratory input with attention to a well defined emergency plan. These patients are in a poor prognostic group.

Further reading

1. Corbridge TC, Hall JB. The assessment and management of adults with status asthmaticus. *American Journal of Respiratory and Critical Care Medicine* 1995; **151**: 1296–316.

2. Guidelines on the management of asthma. Statement by the British Thoracic Society, The British Paediatric Association, the Research Unit of the Royal College of Physicians of London, the King's Fund Centre, the National Asthma Campaign, the Royal College of General Practitioners, the General Practitioners in Asthma Group, The British Association of Accident and Emergency Medicine and the British Paediatric Respiratory Group. *Thorax* 1993; **48**: S1–S24.

3. Garrard CS, Benham S. Bronchodilators in intensive care. In Webb AR, Shapiro MJ, Singer M, Suter P (eds), *Oxford Textbook of Intensive Care*. Oxford: Oxford University Press, 1999: 1241–4.

4. Silverman R. Treatment of acute asthma. A new look at the old and at the new. *Clinics in Chest Medicine* 2000; **21**: 361–79.

5. Leatherman J. Life-threatening asthma. *Clinics in Chest Medicine* 1994; **15**: 453–79.

6. Dhand R, Tobin MJ. Inhaled bronchodilator therapy in mechanically ventilated patients. *American Journal of Respiratory and Critical Care Medicine* 1997; **156**: 3–10.

7. Marquette CH, Saulnier F, Leroy O *et al*. Long-term prognosis of near-fatal asthma. A 6-year follow-up study of 145 asthmatic patients who underwent mechanical ventilation for a near-fatal attack of asthma. *American Journal of Respiratory and Critical Care Medicine* 1992; **146**: 76–81.

17

MANAGEMENT OF COMA CAUSED BY METABOLIC AND ENDOCRINE DYSFUNCTION

G F Mandersloot & D Goldhill

CASE SCENARIO

A 54-year-old woman is admitted to the Accident and Emergency Department after being found unconscious by her daughter. She is an insulin-dependent diabetic who also has treated hypertension. The ambulance paramedics recorded a Glasgow Coma Scale (GCS) score of 3. They administered 20 ml of 50% glucose intravenously, intubated her trachea and started positive-pressure ventilation. On arrival at the hospital, she is hypotensive and hypothermic (33.6°C core temperature) with a blood glucose concentration of 7 mmol.l^{-1}.

DEFINITION AND DESCRIPTION OF THE PROBLEM

Between 3% and 5% of all patients admitted as emergencies to hospital have altered consciousness. Changes range from confusion to coma, with metabolic derangements being the most common cause of non-traumatic coma. Definitions used to describe altered mental states are listed in Table 17.1. A GCS of 8 or less usually indicates coma (Table 17.2).

Although diabetes is an obvious cause of coma in this woman, other possibilities must be considered. Altered consciousness in diabetic patients may arise from hypoglycaemia, ketoacidosis or hyperosmolar non-ketotic abnormalities. An overdose of insulin is a possibility; severe illness, infection, alteration in food and fluid intake, exercise or diarrhoea and vomiting may affect diabetic control. Intracerebral events, such as a stroke, may also precipitate the diabetic crisis; in a hypertensive patient

Table 17.1 – Definitions used to describe the level of consciousness.

Mental state	Definition
Consciousness	Wakefulness with an awareness of self and surroundings
Sleep	A state of mental (and physical) inactivity from which the individual can be aroused
Confusion	Decreased awareness accompanied by disorientation and misinterpretation of the surrounding environment
Delirium	Disorientation in the presence of a state of increased arousal. Irritability, hallucinations or delusions are often present
Stupor	Unresponsive with arousal only possible with vigorous or repeated stimulation
Coma	Unrousable unconsciousness

Table 17.2 – The Glasgow Coma Scale.

Eye opening		Best verbal response		Best motor response	
Clinical sign	Score	Clinical sign	Score	Clinical sign	Score
Spontaneous	4	Oriented	5	Obeys commands	6
To speech	3	Confused	4	Localises to pain	5
To pain	2	Inappropriate	3	Withdraws to pain	4
None	1	Incomprehensible	2	Abnormal flexion	3
		None	1	Extensor response	2
				None	1

GCS is the sum of the individual components: minimum, 3; maximum, 15.

intracranial haemorrhage should be considered. Profound hypothermia will cause coma but may be secondary to other conditions that may themselves depress consciousness levels. These include trauma, poisoning/intoxication or myxoedema. Table 17.3 lists causes of depressed conscious level.

PHYSIOLOGY AND PATHOPHYSIOLOGY

Consciousness can be considered to consist of the interaction of

1. *wakefulness*: a function of the reticular activating system in the midbrain and pons, and

2. *awareness*: a function of the cerebral hemispheres.

The former controls sleep and arousal activity, while the latter is responsible for purposeful cognitive function, for example, motor activity and language. Neither system is independently capable of sustaining consciousness. A wide range of insults, injuries and events can depress conscious levels.

Table 17.3 – Causes of a depressed conscious level.

Lack of substrate and metabolic cofactors
Cerebral anoxia/hypoxia
Hypoglycaemia
Thiamine deficiency and Wernicke's encephalopathy

Organ dysfunction
Hyperglycaemia
Respiratory failure
Renal failure
Hepatic failure
Pancreatitis
Hypopituitarism
Adrenal dysfunction – hyper- and hypoadrenalism
Hypothyroidism (myxoedema)
Hyper- and hypoparathyroidism
Systemic inflammatory response syndrome (e.g. sepsis)
Psychiatric disorders

Electrolyte and acid–base disturbances
Hyper- and hyponatraemia
Hyperosmolar conditions
Hypercalcaemia
Metabolic acidosis and alkalosis

Status epilepticus
Focal or generalised fits

Drugs and toxins
Including alcohol, opioids, tricyclic antidepressants and carbon monoxide poisoning

Body temperature
Hyper- and hypothermia

Intracranial pathology
Stroke
Intracranial haemorrhage
Hydrocephalus
Cerebral oedema
Intracranial tumour, abscess or infection

THERAPEUTIC GOALS

The therapeutic goals in this patient include:

1. Initial resuscitation with stabilisation of vital organ function.

2. Obtaining a history, detailed examination and special investigations.

3. Prevention of secondary brain injury.

4. Identification and treatment of the underlying disorder.

5. Prevention and treatment of complications.

THERAPEUTIC OPTIONS BASED ON PHYSIOLOGICAL AND PHARMACOLOGICAL EFFECTS

The cause of coma is not always immediately evident, and initial management should concentrate on general supportive measures. Assessment of vital organ function should go hand in hand with obtaining a history, detailed examination and special investigations.

Initial resuscitation with stabilisation of vital organ function

Securing a patent airway is of primary importance, followed by restoring adequate oxygen delivery. This nearly always involves providing additional oxygen and, for a comatose patient, will usually require tracheal intubation and positive-pressure ventilation.

Baseline observations and monitoring are an essential and ongoing part of the assessment process. Hypoglycaemia is a common and easily correctable cause of metabolic coma. Early bedside glucose testing will confirm a diagnosis and guide treatment essential to prevent permanent neurological damage.

Obtaining a history, detailed examination and special investigations

History

The history given by relatives, friends, home carers, ambulance crew, or witnesses to the incident can give vital clues to the underlying cause of the coma and as much information as possible should be obtained. Patients with an underlying medical condition such as epilepsy, diabetes mellitus or other endocrine disease, and those taking medication, may wear MedicAlert® bracelets, which may help.

Important factors in the history include:

1.   the exact circumstances surrounding the onset of altered consciousness,

2.   whether the patient is a known epileptic or has suffered from previous convulsions,

3.   whether the patient has suffered previous episodes of loss of consciousness or headaches,

4.   intake of alcohol, drugs or prescription medication, any underlying depressive illness,

5.   history of recent infections, especially those of the upper airway and ears, and

6.   any underlying medical problems, including hypertension, cerebrovascular disease, renal or liver impairment and endocrine abnormalities.

Clinical examination

General examination

Initial examination should start with the assessment of vital signs, including the temperature. Hypothermia often accompanies other medical conditions affecting the central nervous system, and may in itself be responsible for depressing consciousness. Pyrexia is usually present in infection; however, occasionally a raised temperature is of central origin.

Skin colour and changes may point to underlying problems, for example, jaundice in liver failure or a coarse dry skin with hypothyroidism. Evidence of hypodermic injection marks may suggest insulin dependent diabetes mellitus or substance abuse. Petechiae and rashes may suggest an infective cause.

Neurological assessment, examination of the head and neck

An initial assessment of neurological state may be made using the AVPU scale (see Chapter 20). Further detailed neurological examination should include assessment of three main components: conscious level, motor responses and brain stem function. The GCS is used most often to assess the level of mental change (see Table 17.2). Although the GCS was developed to convey information about the level of consciousness and outcome in head injured patients, it is widely used to describe altered consciousness of any origin.

Examination of the motor system may show abnormal posturing, paresis, muscle twitching, and unilateral or bilateral abnormal reflexes. Decerebrate rigidity is seen with upper brain stem lesions, while flaccidity accompanies lower brain stem abnormalities.

When examining the eyes, attention should be paid to the following:

1. *Pupil size*: small, reactive pupils are seen with opioid overdose and hypothalamic or pontine damage, while dilated pupils may be seen with anoxic brain damage or III cranial nerve palsy. Unequally sized pupils may indicate unilateral III cranial nerve compression, but direct trauma to the eye should be excluded.

2. *Response to light*: unreactive pupils are seen in the presence of brain stem or bilateral hemispheric injury, while a unilateral unreactive pupil may follow direct injury. In the majority of metabolic diseases and hemispheric abnormalities, the pupils remain reactive to light.

3. *Reflexes*: corneal as well as oculocephalic and oculovestibular reflexes (assessing brain stem function) may indicate the anatomical structures involved and help quantify the extent of the coma.

4. *Fundi*: evidence of haemorrhage (hypertension or in the presence of a subarachnoid bleed) or retinopathy (diabetic or hypertensive) may give

clues to the underlying diagnosis. With raised intracranial pressure (ICP), papilloedema may be seen.

5. *Cervical spine*: where there is any suspicion of a fall (or other trauma) the cervical spine should be examined for stability. Neck rigidity is most commonly seen in meningial irritation due to subarachnoid haemorrhage or infection, although this may be absent in profound coma.

The skull should always be examined for lacerations and possible underlying fractures. Periorbital (panda eyes) or retroauricular (Battle's sign) haematomas, and spinal fluid rhinorrhoea or otorrhoea are seen with the base of skull fractures.

Respiratory system

Abnormal respiratory patterns are often seen in comatose patients. A raised P_aCO_2 will cause coma. Most causes of coma will result in respiratory depression, which tends to worsen as the depth of coma increases; but tachypnoea may be seen in metabolic acidosis, some head injured patients and poisoning with tricyclic antidepressants or salicylates. Abnormal breathing patterns, such as Cheyne–Stokes respiration or apneustic breathing, are indicative of brain stem dysfunction. Also, when assessing the respiratory system, the smell of alcohol, poisons or ketones may be identified.

Cardiovascular system

Early assessment of heart rate, rhythm, peripheral perfusion and measurement of systemic blood pressure are essential. Arrhythmias may be the result of drug intoxication and could lead to hypotension; atrial fibrillation could indicate embolic disease, while bacterial endocarditis should be considered in the presence of cardiac valvular abnormalities. Hypotension causing low cerebral perfusion can be responsible for an impaired level of consciousness. Therefore, the cause should be identified (invasive monitoring may be helpful) and measures taken to improve circulation.

Abdomen

Palpation of the abdomen may reveal possible underlying medical problems, for example, organomegaly with malignancy, or renal disease such as polycystic kidneys. Abdominal wall rigidity suggests peritoneal irritation and the possibility of sepsis.

Special investigations

The history and clinical examination often provide enough information to make a diagnosis. Further investigations should be directed at the likely cause of the impaired consciousness.

Laboratory investigations

In patients presenting with coma, blood glucose measurement should be performed as a matter of urgency as severe hypoglycaemia (blood glucose $< 1\,\mathrm{mmol.l^{-1}}$) may lead to further neurological damage. Bedside testing should be performed immediately and a sample sent to the laboratory for confirmation. Other tests should include serum urea and electrolytes, arterial blood-gas analysis and full blood count and film. In addition, biochemical tests for liver and endocrine function, urinary electrolytes, glucose and ketones should be performed. Samples (blood, urine and gastric lavage where appropriate) should be examined for toxicology and drug levels. Blood cultures are essential where infection is suspected, as well as in coma of unknown origin. A lumbar puncture is often performed only after CT scanning has ruled out raised ICP. It is an essential investigation where central nervous system infection is suspected.

Neurological imaging

Any neurological imaging should be preceded by adequate resuscitation of vital organ function, since the investigations are performed in isolated areas, and patient access is limited.

(a) *Computed tomography (CT) and magnetic resonance imaging (MRI)*: These imaging methods accurately diagnose space occupying lesions, intracranial haemorrhage and cerebral oedema. Ischaemic lesions and contusions may not always be visible on CT images in the early stages.

(b) *Cerebral angiography*: This is used mainly for the identification and localisation of cerebral aneurysms and arterio-venous malformations.

(c) *Single-photon emission with computed tomography (SPECT) and positron emission tomography (PET)*: These nuclear medicine techniques assess cerebral blood flow and oxygenation, but (currently) have no role in the acute management of metabolic or endocrine-induced coma.

(d) *Skull X-rays*: These are hardly ever informative and only indicated where fractures are suspected.

Electroencephalography (EEG)

The EEG has a limited role in the diagnosis of coma. It may show spikes and sharp wave activity in subclinical status epilepticus (general or focal) and may show abnormal cortical activity in hypoxic brain damage. Evoked potentials could be used to assess the function of specific neurological pathways. However, the EEG and evoked potentials are of little use in prognostication after hypoxic cerebral damage.

Prevention of secondary brain injury

Maintaining adequate cerebral perfusion pressure and cerebral oxygenation is essential to minimise the risk of secondary brain injury. Cerebral perfusion pressure is defined as the mean arterial pressure minus ICP and should be maintained at

60–70 mmHg. Achieving an acceptable cerebral perfusion pressure involves maintaining an adequate mean arterial pressure (often set empirically at 75–80 mmHg, where ICP monitoring is not used) with fluid therapy, vasopressor drugs or inotropic support. The vasoactive drugs used will depend on the clinical picture. Measurement of ICP is indicated in circumstances where the possibility of mass effect and subsequent cerebral herniation exists. Frusemide or mannitol $(0.5–1 \text{ g.kg}^{-1}$ body weight) in repeated doses can be used for the treatment of raised ICP. In these patients, the serum osmolality should be measured. Where the ICP is difficult to control, cerebrospinal fluid drainage via an intraventricular drain can be considered. In addition, reducing the cerebral metabolic rate of oxygen with the use of barbiturates (or propofol) could be considered. The use of moderate hypothermia in these situations, although theoretically beneficial, in clinical practice has not yet been shown to significantly improve outcome.

Correction of hypoglycaemia is essential, but care should be taken since there is some evidence that increased blood glucose levels may worsen cerebral function, especially in ischaemic injury.

Control of convulsions to reduce damage by excessive release of excitatory neurotransmitters such as glutamate is also extremely important. Benzodiazepines (diazepam, lorazepam or midazolam) are most commonly used to terminate convulsions, with phenytoin as second line agent. Barbiturate infusions can be used in resistant cases; EEG monitoring should be used to monitor the pharmacodynamic result. Status epilepticus secondary to a hypoxic cerebral insult may prove very difficult to treat.

Identification and treatment of the underlying disorder

The underlying cause of the coma must be identified. Metabolic and endocrine coma often improves as the underlying medical condition is treated successfully.

Preventive treatment and management of complications

Continuing care should concentrate on the following:

1. ongoing assessment of neurological function;

2. appropriate use of invasive monitoring;

3. nutrition (enteral, if at all possible);

4. stress ulcer prophylaxis where indicated;

5. nursing care with special attention to patient position and pressure areas;

6. physiotherapy (respiratory and limb movement); and

7. prophylaxis, prevention and surveillance for infection.

USUAL OUTCOME

The morbidity and mortality of patients with metabolic and endocrine coma depends on the underlying disorder and severity of secondary cerebral injury. Various markers relating to neurological state, for example, EEG and evoked potential changes, depth of coma and underlying diagnosis have all been used to predict outcome. Coma due to metabolic and endocrine causes and multiple-organ dysfunction have a better outcome than those due to hypoxic or hypotensive insults.

KEY LEARNING POINTS

1. The majority (up to 85%) of non-traumatic coma is metabolic in origin; substance abuse and hypoglycaemia are important causes.

2. Immediate resuscitation of the patient involves securing a patent airway, providing oxygenation and maintaining the circulation.

3. Thorough history taking and examination often give a good indication of the cause of coma and necessary investigations.

4. A high index of suspicion of severe hypoglycaemia as the cause of coma is required; its prompt treatment is essential to prevent further neurological damage.

5. The presence of focal neurological signs warrants early CT or MRI investigation and prompt treatment of raised ICP.

6. Most coma of metabolic or endocrine origin will resolve in due course with the appropriate management of the underlying condition.

Further reading

1. Teasdale G, Jennet B. Assessment of coma and impaired consciousness: a practical scale. *Lancet* 1974; **2**: 81–3.

2. Liu GT. Coma. *Neurosurgery Clinics of North America* 1991; **10**: 579–86.

3. Ashton CH, Teoh R, Davies DM. Drug-induced stupor and coma: some physical signs and their pharmacological basis. *Adverse Drug Reactions and Acute Poisoning Reviews* 1989; **8**: 1–59.

4. Ringel MD. Management of hypothyroidism and hyperthyroidism in the intensive care unit. *Critical Care Clinics* 2001; **17**: 59–74.

5. Quagliarello VJ, Scheld M. Treatment of bacterial meningitis. *New England Journal of Medicine* 1997; **336**: 708–16.

6. Heafield MTE. Managing status epilepticus. *British Medical Journal* 2000; **320**: 953–4.

7. Qureshi AI, Tuhrim S, Broderick JP, Batjer HH, Hondo H, Hanley DF. Spontaneous intracerebral hemorrhage. *New England Journal of Medicine* 2001; **344**: 1450–60.

8. Goldhill DR. Post-resuscitation intensive care. In Goldhill DR, Withington S (eds), *Textbook of Intensive Care*. London: Chapman and Hall, 1996: 27–32.

9. Riordan SM, Williams R. Treatment of hepatic encephalopathy. *New England Journal of Medicine* 1997; **337**: 473–9.

18

MANAGEMENT OF STATUS EPILEPTICUS AND PYREXIA

S J MacKenzie

CASE SCENARIO

A 20-year-old man is brought to the Accident and Emergency (A&E) Department following a grand mal seizure in the street. On arrival, 20 min after the onset, he remains in status epilepticus. He is treated with two 10 mg boluses of intravenous diazepam with good effect, but the seizures recur. He continues to fit despite the administration of further intravenous diazepam (10 mg) and an intravenous infusion of phenytoin ($20\,mg.kg^{-1}$); the seizures are finally controlled with a propofol infusion ($4\,mg.kg^{-1}.h^{-1}$). His trachea is intubated and mechanical ventilation is started in the A&E Department before transfer to the intensive care unit (ICU). He requires cardiovascular support with fluids and dobutamine ($7.5\,\mu g.kg^{-1}.min^{-1}$) and has a central line inserted. After 24 h, he develops a pyrexia due to aspiration pneumonia and broad spectrum antibiotics are prescribed. He responds well to treatment and his pyrexia initially settles but recurs after 1 week.

DEFINITION AND DESCRIPTION OF THE PROBLEM

Status epilepticus

Status epilepticus is continuous or intermittent seizures without recovery of consciousness. Sometimes the definition includes a reference to seizure duration of approximately 20–30 min, but 5 min seizure activity is sufficient to make the diagnosis.

Status epilepticus is usually easy to recognise in the early stages, but muscle twitching may be subtle and tends to become less prominent with time. True, non-convulsive status epilepticus can occur and is easily missed. It should be included in the

Table 18.1 – Possible causes of status epilepticus.

Pre-existing epilepsy, particularly if drug treatment has recently been altered or compliance is poor
Cerebral tumours
Stroke (ischaemic or haemorrhagic)
Intracranial infection
Hypoxic brain damage
Drug toxicity (including therapeutic toxicity and intentional overdose)
Electrolyte disturbances (hyponatraemia, hypocalcaemia and hypomagnesaemia)
Hypoglycaemia

differential diagnosis of unexplained coma. The differential diagnosis of status epilepticus includes rigors, myoclonic jerking, generalised dystonia and pseudo-status. The latter may occur in known epileptics and, on occasion, may be very difficult to distinguish from true status. An electroencephalograph (EEG) may be required to differentiate the two.

Between 102 000 and 152 000 cases of status epilepticus occur annually in the United States. In 50% of cases, the patient is not previously known to be epileptic. Some of these will be first presentations of idiopathic epilepsy but most will have an underlying cause (Table 18.1). Critically ill patients without epilepsy are also at increased risk of seizures including status.

The mortality associated with status epilepticus is approximately 25%, but most deaths are due to the underlying cause rather than the seizures themselves. Generally, patients with chronic processes are more likely to respond to treatment. The longer seizure activity persists, the greater the risk of neurological damage and the lower the chance that treatment will be effective. Status epilepticus is therefore a medical emergency.

Pyrexia

Pyrexia, defined as a core temperature greater than 38.3°C, is a common, but non-specific, finding which may be insignificant or may indicate serious illness. The use of paracetamol or extra-corporeal circuits may mask pyrexia.

PATHOLOGY AND PATHOPHYSIOLOGY

Status epilepticus may be due to excessive excitation or deficient inhibition of cerebral neurones, and there is some evidence that antagonism of the neurotransmitter γ-aminobutyric acid (GABA) or alterations to $GABA_A$ receptors may be involved.

Cerebral effects of status epilepticus

The most important consequence of status epilepticus is cerebral damage. This is due to a combination of direct and systemic effects. Seizures cause release of glutamate, which activates post-synaptic glutamate receptors, allowing calcium to enter cells. The rise in intracellular calcium concentration and resulting enzyme activation is responsible for cellular damage. Seizure activity lasting over 30 min is likely to cause permanent damage to cerebral structures, particularly the hippocampus. Consequently, merely controlling the physical manifestation of seizures will not prevent neurological damage.

Seizures are also associated with an increased cerebral metabolic rate, which can be met initially by a reflex increase in cerebral blood flow. However, failure of cerebral autoregulation leads to reduced cerebral blood flow and increased intracranial pressure.

Peripheral effects of status epilepticus

Status epilepticus affects the cardiovascular, respiratory, renal and musculoskeletal systems. Important sequelae of status include airway obstruction, loss of protective reflexes in the airway and reduced ventilation. There will be an associated increase in oxygen consumption. Pyrexia and metabolic acidosis are likely to be due to increased muscle and autonomic activity, but persistent pyrexia may indicate an underlying infection. Infection may be the primary cause of status, and pulmonary aspiration a potential consequence. The phase of increased autonomic activity may also produce arrhythmias and neurogenic pulmonary oedema. Infrequently, rhabdomyolysis may cause renal failure.

Causes of pyrexia

There are many causes of pyrexia, including infection, central pyrexia, acalculous cholecystitis, pancreatitis, bowel ischaemia, myocardial infarction, pulmonary embolism and reactions to drugs, blood and blood products. Fever due to drugs, including antibiotics, antifungals and phenytoin, may not immediately follow administration and need not be accompanied by either a rash or eosinophilia.

Consequences of pyrexia

The development of a fever facilitates the immune response; it may also inhibit bacterial and viral replication. Heart rate, metabolic rate and CO_2 production increase but the extent to which these are due to the underlying cause rather than simply the temperature is uncertain.

THERAPEUTIC GOALS

The therapeutic goals dictate that:

1. Seizures should be abolished as rapidly as possible. Early treatment minimises the risk of neural damage and is more likely to be successful. Measures to prevent further seizures should be taken.

2. Remediable causes should be corrected.

3. The airway and cardio-respiratory complications of seizures and of their treatment should be urgently addressed.

4. The causes of pyrexia should be sought and appropriate therapy commenced.

THERAPEUTIC OPTIONS BASED ON PHYSIOLOGICAL AND PHARMACOLOGICAL EFFECTS

The initial management of status epilepticus focuses on ensuring control of the airway, breathing and circulation, with rapid termination of seizures.

Control of seizures and prevention of recurrence

While attention must be paid to reversible causes of seizures (e.g. hypoglycaemia, hyponatraemia), most patients will require anticonvulsant therapy. Recent data suggest that lorazepam is the anticonvulsant of choice for initial management.

Benzodiazepines

Benzodiazepines are GABA agonists; they may also produce a phenytoin-like inhibition of repetitive neuronal firing at higher doses. Their rapid action makes them useful in first line treatment of status epilepticus. Intravenous lorazepam $0.1 \, mg.kg^{-1}$ is preferable to diazepam, as it has a longer duration of action (12–24 h compared to 15–30 min) making recurrence less likely. Lorazepam has the theoretical disadvantage of a slower onset of action. All benzodiazepines depress conscious level and can cause both respiratory and cardiac depression. Rectal diazepam can be given by ambulance paramedics or relatives, but is not frequently used in hospital.

Phenytoin and fosphenytoin

An intravenous infusion of phenytoin ($15–20 \, mg.kg^{-1}$ over approximately 20 min) can be used as a first line agent in status epilepticus but, because lorazepam is probably more effective and acts quicker, phenytoin should really be regarded as second line treatment. Higher doses are sometimes required and plasma concentrations may need to exceed the 'therapeutic range' ($10–20 \, mg.l^{-1}$).

Phenytoin can cause hypotension and cardiac dysrhythmias. Consequently, the maximum rate of infusion is $50 \, mg.min^{-1}$, which delays its onset of action. Phenytoin is irritant and should be given into a large vein. It may cause phlebitis and severe tissue necrosis ('purple glove syndrome'). Such complications can be minimised if fosphenytoin, a water soluble pro-drug, is used. Whenever phenytoin or fosphenytoin are administered by infusion, ECG monitoring is essential.

Other anticonvulsants

Phenobarbital ($10–20 \, mg.kg^{-1}$) is effective but its side effects (e.g. respiratory depression, hypotension and prolonged sedation) limit its use to patients in whom benzodiazepines and phenytoin have failed. The intravenous or rectal administration of paraldehyde remains a valuable adjunct for managing status, especially outside hospital. Sodium valproate has been reported to be effective and is now available for intravenous use.

Propofol and thiopentone

The use of general anaesthesia is invaluable for managing resistant status epilepticus. Thiopentone has a rapid onset of action, but brain concentrations fall quickly due to redistribution so that maintenance requires an infusion. When given by infusion, both thiopentone and its active metabolites accumulate, producing prolonged sedation which interferes with subsequent neurological assessment. Thiopentone is immuno-suppressive and increases the risk of nosocomial infection.

Propofol also has a rapid onset of action but a much shorter recovery period, as it does not accumulate when given by infusion. Despite animal studies suggesting that it can be proconvulsant and reports of seizures associated with its use during anaesthesia, propofol is preferred to thiopentone in many ICUs. Ideally, the dose of propofol should not exceed $5\,\mathrm{mg.kg^{-1}.h^{-1}}$. Both propofol and thiopentone cause hypotension, making cardiovascular support necessary.

When giving either agent, it is highly desirable to employ continuous processed EEG monitoring as seizures may be present with no or almost undetectable motor activity. It is traditional to titrate anticonvulsant therapy to produce burst suppression or even iso-electric patterns; however, this is not necessary provided seizures are controlled. Treatment should continue for 24 h following the last seizure. General anaesthesia is instituted when patients are resistant to other treatment but it is important that more conventional anticonvulsants are continued in order to reduce the chance of recurrence when the general anaesthetic is stopped.

Neuromuscular blockers

Neuromuscular blockers have no role in the management of status epilepticus, except to facilitate tracheal intubation. Paralysis does not prevent neural damage due to persistent seizures but does prevent clinical detection. In the very unusual case where neuromuscular blockade is required for a patient with status (e.g. acute respiratory distress syndrome due to aspiration pneumonia producing severe hypoxaemic respiratory failure), EEG monitoring is essential.

Investigation and treatment of the cause of seizures

It is important to obtain a patient history at an early stage; relatives, witnesses, the general practitioner and previous hospital records may all be helpful. Useful investigations in the search for potentially reversible causes for seizures include a full blood count, urea, electrolytes and plasma glucose measurement, arterial blood gas analysis and, for known epileptics, serum anticonvulsant levels.

If the blood sugar concentration is below $2.5\,mmol.l^{-1}$, intravenous dextrose (50 ml of 50% solution) should be administered. Empirical use of concentrated dextrose solutions is not advised, since hyperglycaemia will exacerbate cerebral damage. If there is any suspicion of alcoholism, thiamine should also be given.

Central nervous system (CNS) infections are a less common cause of fits than intracerebral tumour or stroke; consequently, a CT scan of the brain should be performed before a lumbar puncture. Raised intracranial pressure is common after seizures and may also occur with CNS infection. The risks and benefits of lumbar puncture must be considered on an individual basis, but antibiotic treatment should not be delayed. An elevated white cell count in the cerebrospinal fluid (CSF) may be caused by seizures and is not conclusive evidence of infection.

Prevention and treatment of complications

Pulmonary aspiration, due to depressed laryngeal reflexes, is a serious risk during seizures, and tracheal intubation may be required to protect the airway. Seizure activity is usually accompanied initially by hyperventilation but respiration is often depressed later due to a combination of the disease and the treatment. Cardiac depression is usually due to the effects of therapy or, occasionally, hypoxaemia. Patients admitted with status epilepticus are vulnerable to the same complications of ICU admission as other patients, and one of these is the later development of pyrexia.

Pyrexia

The priority here is to establish and treat the cause. Although pyrexia is a very common feature of acute illness, especially in critically ill patients, there is little evidence that, *per se*, it requires treatment in adults. Possible exceptions include patients with raised intracranial pressure, intractable hypoxaemia or persistent hypercapnia, where a raised temperature may be disadvantageous. Paradoxically, attempts at external cooling may raise the core temperature.

The initial step in diagnosis is to rule out the possibility of infection, using clinical and laboratory tests. Common infections in critically ill patients include pneumonia, urinary tract infections, wound infections, intravascular catheter related sepsis, peritonitis and sinusitis. If the cause is not obvious, two or three sets of blood cultures should be obtained from separate skin puncture sites; samples of sputum and urine, and wound swabs should be sent for microbiological analysis. CSF analysis may also be required. Specimens should be examined without delay, as some organisms die rapidly.

Colonisation and infection are common in the ICU and can be very difficult to distinguish. Infection, particularly due to fungi, may exist when cultures are negative. Total and differential white cell count, C-reactive protein and procalcitonin levels have all been suggested as specific markers of infection, but none reliably discriminates infected from non-infected patients. However, they may be valuable in monitoring response to treatment. Empirical treatment with antibiotics must often commence before laboratory diagnosis is available, particularly, in patients who are neutropoenic or immuno-compromised.

Common infections in the intensive care patient

A 1 day point prevalence study of European ICUs in 1992 found that 45% of ICU patients were infected and that 21% had acquired infection while in the ICU. The common sites and organisms are shown in Table 18.2.

Table 18.2 – Frequency of ICU acquired infections.

(a) Site	
Pneumonia	47%
Lower respiratory tract (not pneumonia)	18%
Urinary tract	18%
Blood (laboratory confirmed)	12%
Wound	7%
Ear, nose and throat	5%
(b) Organisms	
Enterobacteriaceae (*Escherichia coli, Klebsiella and Enterobacter*)	34%
Staphylococcus aureus	30%
Pseudomonas	29%
Coagulase negative staphylococci	19%
Fungi	17%

Modified from Vincent J-L, Bihari DJ, Suter PM *et al*. The prevalence of nosocomial infection in ICUs in Europe. *Journal of the American Medical Association* 1995; 274: 639–44. Some patients had more than one site or organism.

The resurgence of gram-positive organisms has continued, and there has been an increase in antibiotic resistance amongst *Staphylococcus aureus, Enterococci, Pseudomonas* and *Acinetobacter*. Fungal infection is also an increasing concern. Effective empirical treatment requires knowledge of local patterns of infection and bacterial resistance. An apparently new infection may actually be a recurrence of original infection due to ineffective treatment.

Community acquired pneumonia

This accounts for a significant proportion of ICU admissions. In addition to tracheal aspirates or bronchoalveolar lavage specimens, blood should be sent for microbiological culture and pneumococcal antigen detection. A urine sample should be analysed for legionella titres. Empirical treatment (e.g. cefuroxime and erythromycin) should take account of known local prevalence but must cover *Streptococcus pneumonia*, which still accounts for 60–70% of cases. If pneumococcal infection is confirmed, benzylpenicillin is still considered the drug of choice, although resistance is increasing.

Ventilator associated pneumonia

Ventilator associated pneumonia (VAP) develops more than 48–72 h after starting mechanical ventilation. The source may be endogenous (secondary to colonisation of the oropharynx) or exogenous (i.e. cross-infection). The most common organisms are *Enterobacter* or *Staphylococcus aureus*. A number of features may suggest the development of VAP, namely new fever, increase in purulent bronchial secretions, deterioration in blood gas exchange, elevated (or depressed) white cell count, or new findings on clinical examination or chest X-ray. Confirming the diagnosis and distinguishing colonisation from infection may be very difficult. Bronchoalveolar lavage or protected brush specimens may be desirable but are not easily undertaken routinely. Semi-quantitative culture of tracheal aspirates is useful. Microscopy will help to differentiate saliva, where epithelial cells will be present, from lower respiratory tract specimens; gram staining is helpful in categorising the infecting organism.

Catheter related infections

Any intravascular catheter may be a source of infection, but central venous and pulmonary artery catheters (PACs) are most frequently responsible. The most common organisms are Staphylococci and Enterococci.

Lines may be infected at the time of insertion if aseptic techniques are poor. Those which are inserted in an emergency without full asepsis should be changed as soon as the patient is stable. Later infection may occur via the ports, the catheter insertion site or haematogenous spread, especially if there is thrombus on the catheter. The risk of systemic infection with PACs rises with time and they should be removed within 72 h of insertion unless their continued use is deemed clinically essential. Antibiotic impregnated catheters probably reduce the incidence of line sepsis.

Timely diagnosis of line related sepsis is difficult. Where the patient is stable, it may be safe to swab insertion sites and take blood for quantitative culture from both the lines and peripheral blood. If the colony count from the line cultures is greater than five times the culture from peripheral blood, line associated infection is likely. If line related sepsis is strongly suspected, line removal is indicated, recognising that only 15–26% of lines removed for this reason are confirmed as infected. Some prefer to change lines over a guide wire and then culture the line, but this carries a high risk of re-infection.

Methicillin resistant Staphylococcus aureus

Methicillin resistant *Staphylococcus aureus* (MRSA) is endemic in many hospitals. Where colonisation with MRSA occurs, careful attention should be paid to infection control measures. However, definite MRSA infection requires aggressive antibiotic therapy using vancomycin, teicoplanin or linezolid. Vancomycin can cause renal failure and plasma levels should be monitored regularly.

USUAL OUTCOME

The outcome from status epilepticus is usually good but depends on the underlying cause. Provided that the patient reaches hospital (or has seizures controlled) within 30 min, death or serious disability from status or its immediate complications is unusual. However, if status epilepticus is the expression of a catastrophic neurological event, outcome will be influenced by the prognosis of the underlying condition.

Similarly, pyrexia is not generally fatal in itself, and outcome depends on the cause. Pyrexia occurring after several days in ICU is most likely to be due to nosocomial infection. Nosocomial infection is more common in sicker patients, who are already at high risk of death. Therefore, the direct impact of nosocomial infection on mortality is difficult to quantify, although it is suggested that it may increase it by up to 30%.

KEY LEARNING POINTS

1. Seizures lasting 20–30 min are likely to cause permanent neurological damage.

2. Mortality in status epilepticus is related to the cause.

3. Lorazepam is the drug of choice for the initial treatment of status epilepticus.

4. If propofol or thiopentone are required, other anticonvulsants should be continued and EEG monitoring employed.

5. Neuromuscular blocking agents should not be used in status epilepticus, except to facilitate tracheal intubation or to treat refractory hypoxaemia. EEG monitoring is then essential.

6. Pyrexia does not necessarily indicate infection.

7. Pyrexia should not normally be treated in adults.

8. Nosocomial infection is common in the ICU and is often due to multiple organisms, which may be resistant to antibiotics. A rational and systematic approach to diagnosis and treatment of nosocomial infection requires local microbiological data.

Further reading

1. Lowenstein DH, Alldredge BK. Status epilepticus. *New England Journal of Medicine* 1998; **338**: 970–6.

2. Delanty N, Vaughan CJ, French JA. Medical causes of seizures. *Lancet* 1998; **352**: 383–90.

3. O'Grady NP, Barie PS, Bartlett JG *et al.* Practice guidelines for evaluating new fever in critically ill adult patients. *Clinical Infectious Diseases* 1998; **26**: 1042–59.

4. Treiman DM, Meyers PD, Walton NY *et al.* A comparison of four treatments for generalised convulsive status epilepticus. *New England Journal of Medicine* 1998; **338**: 792–8.

5. Llewelyn M, Cohen J. Diagnosis of infection in sepsis. *Intensive Care Medicine* 2001; **27**: S10–S32.

6. Vincent J-L, Mercan D. Dear Sirs, What is your PCT? *Intensive Care Medicine* 2000; **26**: 1170–1.

7. Vincent J-L, Bihari DJ, Suter PM *et al.* The prevalence of nosocomial infection in intensive care units in Europe. *Journal of the American Medical Association* 1995; **274**: 639–44.

19

CRUSH AND SPINAL INJURIES CAUSED BY AN INDUSTRIAL ACCIDENT

R Craven & J Nolan

CASE SCENARIO

A 42-year-old man is injured when scaffolding collapses under him. He falls 15 ft and is trapped by scaffolding and rubble across his legs. He is initially unconscious at the scene, but recovers rapidly. After 2 h he is released and

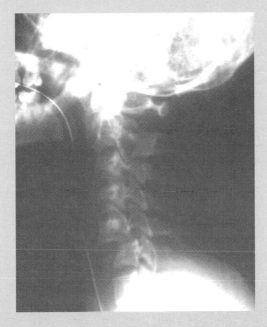

Lateral radiograph of the cervical spine showing subluxation of C5 on C6. This is an inadequate view because it does not include the upper part of the first thoracic vertebra.

brought to the Accident and Emergency (A&E) Department. On arrival, his airway is clear and his respiratory rate is 30 breaths.min^{-1}. While receiving oxygen 15 l.min^{-1} via a face mask with a reservoir, his arterial oxygen saturation by pulse oximetry is 97%. His blood pressure is 76/40 mmHg and pulse rate is 46 beats.min^{-1}. He has a large bruise on his occiput, but is awake with a Glasgow Coma Scale (GCS) score of 14. The blood pressure improves to 100/40 mmHg after an infusion of 2.5 l of normal saline. His left thigh and both legs below the knees are deformed and tensely swollen. He is unable to move his legs and has very weak arms. Radiographs of the chest and pelvis are normal. A lateral cervical spine radiograph shows a 60% subluxation of the vertebral body of C5 on C6 (see figure above).

Radiographs of the lower limbs show a comminuted fracture of the left femur and fractures of both tibias and fibulae.

DEFINITION AND DESCRIPTION OF THE PROBLEM

Spinal injuries are an important cause of long-term disability after trauma. The most common cause of traumatic spinal injury is road traffic accidents (52%) followed by industrial and domestic accidents (27%), and then sporting accidents (16%). Up to 5% of patients with major trauma have unstable cervical spine injuries, and one third of these are associated with neurological deficit. While little can be done about the primary injury, secondary injury must be prevented. All patients with serious injuries, and those with neurological signs or symptoms or a reduced level of consciousness have the potential for spinal injury and their spines should be immobilised.

The most common regions of the spine to be damaged are those that are most mobile, namely the cervical spine and the thoracolumbar junction. In adults, the lower cervical spine is most commonly affected, while in children it is the upper cervical spine. Unstable injuries involving the thoracic spine are uncommon, because the spine is stabilised by the rib cage.

Crush injuries typically involve the lower limbs and may cause compartment syndrome and rhabdomyolysis. Serious crush injuries can occur in the absence of fractures. A high index of suspicion is needed to detect compartment syndrome and rhabdomyolysis. Early diagnosis and appropriate intervention will reduce morbidity and mortality.

PATHOLOGY AND PATHOPHYSIOLOGY

Spinal injuries

The spinal cord may be affected by primary and/or secondary injury. Primary spinal injury occurs at the time of the accident when extreme flexion, extension or rotation causes fractures or ligamentous disruption of the spinal column and stretching of the spinal cord. The cord can be injured by direct compression from bone fragments and foreign bodies. Primary injury may also be caused by ischaemia, if the vertebral arteries or the branches of the thoracolumbar aorta that form the anterior spinal artery are disrupted. After the initial injury, local tissue hypoxia produces a neurochemical cascade causing the release of neural proteases, free radicals and a rise in intra-cellular calcium leading to cell death.

Once the primary injury has occurred, secondary injury may follow. This is caused by progressive cord oedema, hypoxaemia and hypotension, all of which will exacerbate the local tissue hypoxia and accelerate and extend the area of cell death.

Injury to the spinal cord will affect many of the body's systems depending on the level of injury.

Respiratory system

The degree of respiratory insufficiency depends on the level of the cord damage and associated injuries. Spinal cord oedema causes the level of the injury to ascend; these changes are maximal at 72 h.

Spinal cord injury above C4 causes loss of all intercostal and diaphragmatic function. Accessory muscle function may also be lost and these patients will require immediate intubation. Injury at the C4–C5 level causes loss of all intercostal function and reduced diaphragmatic function, but the accessory muscles are intact. Vital capacity is reduced to 20–25% of normal and the respiratory pattern is one of diaphragmatic breathing. These patients will need ventilatory support, at least in the early stages. Below the C5 level, accessory and diaphragmatic function is intact, but there may be variable loss of intercostal function depending on the exact level of injury.

Cardiovascular system

Most patients with high spinal injury are initially hypotensive because of both hypovolaemia and spinal shock. Spinal shock occurs in cord injuries above the T1 level due to vasodilatation from the loss of sympathetic outflow and bradycardia from loss of the cardiac accelerator fibres (T1–T5). Lesions below this level cause variable loss of sympathetic outflow with vasodilatation below the level of the lesion and compensatory vasoconstriction above, leading to maintenance of blood pressure. In all cases, there is impairment of compensatory mechanisms for blood-pressure control; haemorrhage or postural changes are tolerated poorly. Loss of the sympathetic supply allows unopposed vagal action, so that any stimuli to the vagus, such as suction or catheterisation, can cause bradycardia.

In all cases of trauma, including those with spinal damage, it is essential to exclude haemorrhagic shock. For example, the symptoms and signs of intra-abdominal bleeding, such as pain and tenderness or tachycardia, may be masked by the spinal injury.

Nervous system

Below the level of the lesion there is flaccid paralysis, with loss of both autonomic and motor reflexes, and loss of sensation. Sacral sparing indicates an incomplete spinal cord lesion with the potential for good recovery. The stage of flaccid paralysis may last for up to 6 weeks before gradually being replaced by spasticity. Suxamethonium should be avoided from 3 days after injury, because stimulation of denervated muscle, in which acetylcholine receptors have proliferated, may cause massive release of potassium.

Genitourinary system

Bladder atony causes incomplete emptying or urinary retention.

Gastrointestinal system

Gastric dilatation and paralytic ileus increase the risk of pulmonary aspiration.

Thermoregulation

Loss of sympathetic supply impairs cutaneous vasoconstriction, dilatation and sweating; the patient becomes poikilothermic.

Crush injuries

Muscle damage can occur after all types of trauma, but it is particularly common after entrapment under rubble or in vehicles. Myocyte necrosis causes release of myoglobin, creatinine kinase (CK) and other cellular contents. Rhabdomyolysis can cause acute renal failure, compartment syndrome and derangements of plasma calcium and phosphate.

The diagnosis of rhabdomyolysis is made when serum CK exceeds $600\,\text{i.u.}\cdot\text{l}^{-1}$ or six times the upper limit of normal. Severe crush injury will result in a CK level of many thousands. The CK begins to rise 2–12 h after injury and reaches a peak at 1–3 days.

Acute renal failure

Rhabdomyolysis causes renal failure by three mechanisms:

1. *Tubular obstruction*: myoglobin precipitates in the renal tubules; cast formation is enhanced by acidic conditions and poor washout.

2. *Tubular damage by oxidant injury*: the haem group of myoglobin causes lipid peroxidation, particularly in the proximal tubule.

3. *Vasoconstriction*: movement of fluid into damaged muscle causes hypovolaemia and reduced renal blood flow.

Compartment syndrome

As the injured myocytes swell, the intra-compartmental pressure rises rapidly in those muscle groups confined within tight fibrous sheaths (e.g. calf, forearm, foot, hand, gluteal region and thigh). When the compartment pressure exceeds venous pressure, capillary blood flow is impaired causing muscle ischaemia and, eventually, necrosis. The pressure at which this occurs is approximately 30–40 mmHg, but it can be lower if the systemic blood pressure is also low. The signs and symptoms of compartment syndrome are:

1. pain, which is made worse by passive stretching of the involved muscles;

2. paraesthesiae;

3. decreased sensation;

4. tense swelling of the involved compartment; and

5. weakness or paralysis of involved muscles.

The loss of peripheral pulses is a late sign of compartment syndrome.

Electrolyte complications

The release of myocyte contents causes hyperkalaemia, hyperphosphataemia, hypo-calcaemia and metabolic acidosis. Sodium and water enters the myocytes from the extracellular compartment, which contributes to hypovolaemia. Initially, rhabdo-myolysis causes hypocalcaemia as calcium enters the injured myocyte. Later, hyper-calcaemia can develop as parathyroid hormone levels increase and calcium leaves the cells.

THERAPEUTIC GOALS

The goals for spinal injury include:

1. Prevention of cord damage by early and complete immobilisation of the spinal column and log rolling techniques.

2. Aggressive resuscitation with attention to airway, breathing and circulation to prevent secondary injury.

3. Recognition and treatment of associated injuries.

4. Prevention and treatment of the early and late complications of spinal injury.

The goals for crush injuries include:

1. Initiation of adequate fluid resuscitation to restore normovolaemia and maintain a good urine output.

2. Early diagnosis and treatment of compartment syndrome.

3. Treatment of the metabolic derangements caused by rhabdomyolysis.

4. Provision of renal support.

THERAPEUTIC OPTIONS BASED ON PHYSIOLOGICAL AND PHARMACOLOGICAL EFFECTS

Spinal injuries

Immobilisation

Early and complete spinal immobilisation will reduce movement of the vertebral column and minimise further damage to the spinal cord. The patient should be transferred to the hospital on a spinal board with full cervical immobilisation using a rigid collar, lateral blocks and strong tape across the forehead and chin. On arrival at the hospital, the patient should be moved from the spinal board as soon as possible, as patients with spinal cord injury develop decubitus ulcers very rapidly. A log rolling technique should be used to turn the patient.

Airway

The airway may be compromised by a reduced level of consciousness secondary to head injuries, hypoxaemia or hypotension or because of facial injuries. Intubation may be necessary either to secure the airway or to aid ventilation in high spinal injuries. There is debate over the best method of intubating the patient with a cervical spine injury. The main options are:

1. pre-oxygenation, manual in-line stabilisation of the cervical spine, application of cricoid pressure, intravenous induction of anaesthesia and paralysis with suxamethonium, direct laryngoscopy and oral intubation;

2. awake fibreoptic intubation under topical or local anaesthesia.

It is extremely unlikely that properly controlled intubation of patients with unstable spines will cause further spinal cord injury, but untreated hypotension following induction of anaesthesia can cause cord injury. The choice of intubation technique is determined by urgency and the skill of the operator. In the resuscitation room, direct laryngoscopy and oral intubation is usually preferred. Manual in-line stabilisation of the cervical spine restricts the view of the epiglottis at laryngoscopy. Consequently, the need to use a gum elastic bougie and/or McCoy laryngoscope should be anticipated.

Breathing

Oxygen should be administered to the patient by face mask and the arterial oxygen saturation monitored by pulse oximetry. The level of spinal injury and associated injuries will determine the need for assisted ventilation.

Circulation

Hypovolaemia can be secondary to both haemorrhage and spinal shock. Resuscitation with crystalloid is usually sufficient to reverse the hypotension of spinal shock. If not, the alpha agonist metaraminol ($20-50 \mu g.min^{-1}$) should be used to achieve an adequate spinal cord perfusion pressure ($\approx$70 mmHg). Autoregulation of spinal cord blood flow is disrupted after injury and the therapeutic concepts are the same as those applied to the treatment of cerebral injury. Assuming a moderately elevated cerebrospinal fluid pressure, a mean arterial pressure of 90 mmHg should result in a spinal cord perfusion pressure of at least 70 mmHg. Patients with spinal injuries are prone to pulmonary oedema, because massive sympathetic outflow at the time of injury causes transient systemic and pulmonary hypertension, leading to pulmonary capillary disruption. A pulmonary artery catheter can be helpful when hypotension persists despite adequate fluid resuscitation and the exclusion of occult haemorrhage. Atropine may be required to prevent the profound bradycardia often provoked by coughing or suctioning.

Disability

If possible, the extent of any neurological deficit should be assessed before sedation and intubation.

Exposure

The patient should be log rolled in order to assess the back for bruising, steps, swelling, pain and to examine the tone of the anal sphincter. For an adult patient, this requires one person to control the head and cervical spine, three people to roll, and a fifth to examine the patient. Patients with cervical spinal injuries are unable to regulate their body temperature effectively and care must be taken to avoid hypothermia.

Adjunctive treatment

Provided there is no evidence of a basal skull fracture, a nasogastric tube should be inserted as spinal injury patients commonly develop acute gastric dilatation. If untreated, this may increase the risk of regurgitation and aspiration, and/or compromise ventilation by splinting of the diaphragm. If the patient is intubated, an oro-gastric tube may be used. A urinary catheter should be inserted, as urinary retention is common; urine output must be monitored closely.

Specific treatment

The National Acute Spinal Cord Injury Study (NASCIS) II and III trials appear to demonstrate a small improvement in maximal motor recovery when patients are given steroids within 8 h of a spinal cord injury. In accordance with the NASCIS trials, an initial intravenous bolus of methylprednisolone 30 mg.kg^{-1} should be given over 15 min, followed 45 min later by an infusion of 5.4 mg.kg^{-1} over the next 23 h if started within 3 h of injury, and for 47 h if started 3–8 h after injury. However, many clinicians, particularly in the UK, are unconvinced by the reported benefits of steroids and consider the increased risk of sepsis to be unacceptable.

Spinal clearance

Further imaging of the spine should be undertaken after life threatening injuries have been treated. Spinal clearance requires adequate radiographic views combined with a thorough clinical examination. The British Trauma Society has recently produced guidelines on clearing the spine (Figure 19.1).

A reliable clinical examination can be made only if the patient is conscious, unimpaired by drugs or alcohol and has no distracting injuries that will mask pain from the spine. As a minimum, there must be lateral (C1 to top of T1), anteroposterior and odontoid peg radiographs of the cervical spine and lateral and anteroposterior views of the thoracolumbar spine. CT scanning with reconstruction to view any part of the spine not seen clearly on plain radiographs should be used. The inability to reliably examine the unconscious patient makes clearing the spine difficult. Plain radiography and CT scanning can miss significant ligamentous injuries unaccompanied by subluxation or fracture. These injuries are extremely rare, but uncontrolled movement of the patient could cause cord damage and, for this reason, many clinicians will not clear the spine until the patient is conscious and able to comply with a physical examination. The rigid cervical collar should be removed to prevent pressure sores, but lateral head supports are left in position and log rolling is continued. The problem with this approach is that turning the patient requires several nurses, and prolonged periods in the supine position increases the risk of pneumonia. Other approaches to clearing the unconscious patient's spine include:

1. Continuous X-ray screening of the cervical spine, while it is moved through full flexion and extension; this requires very experienced personnel and is not risk free.

2. Use of magnetic resonance imaging to exclude ligamentous injury and lesions to the cord.

3. Reliance on radiographs and CT scans alone. Many physicians adopt the pragmatic view that plain radiography of the spine, combined with CT scanning of those parts of the spine not seen well on radiographs, should be enough for experienced clinicians to 'clear' the spine and allow unrestricted nursing and turning.

Surgical treatment

The aim of surgical treatment is to reduce and stabilise unstable fractures and so prevent further cord damage. Management may be either conservative (i.e. traction via skull tongs or a halo frame) or surgical (i.e. open reduction and internal fixation).

Intensive care complications

Respiratory complications leading to pneumonia are the most common cause of death in patients with spinal injuries. Aggressive physiotherapy and respiratory muscle training are important to avoid intubation. Ventilatory support will be necessary if the vital capacity is below $10\,ml.kg^{-1}$. Tracheostomy is commonly required in those needing prolonged ventilatory support or who have a very weak

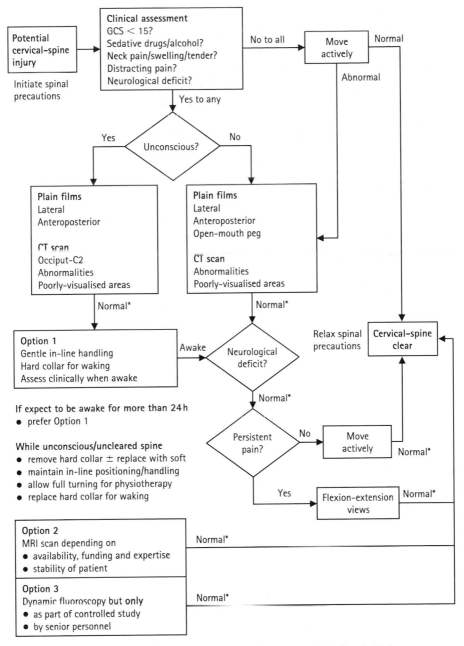

Figure 19.1 – The British Trauma Society Cervical Spinal Clearance Algorithm (courtesy: Dr Peter Oakley).

cough. Respiratory function tends to improve as the flaccid paralysis changes to spasticity.

The initial spinal shock gradually resolves, but patients continue to have a low normal pulse rate and blood pressure. Patients with lesions above the T7 level may exhibit the autonomic mass effect (i.e. intermittent hypertension with bradycardia and sweating). This is caused by triggering of a spinal sympathetic reflex, which is normally inhibited from above. Massive vasoconstriction below the level of the lesion provokes a vagal response and vasodilation above the injury. Classic triggers are overdistension of the bladder or rectum.

Gastrointestinal complications include stress ulceration, which is reduced by early enteral feeding or, if this is not tolerated, by the use of H_2-antagonists or sucralfate. Paralytic ileus is common and prokinetics and laxatives may be necessary.

Patients with spinal injuries commonly develop deep vein thrombosis and pulmonary embolism (5% within 2–3 weeks). Anti-embolic stockings should be applied and subcutaneous low molecular weight heparin administered.

Meticulous nursing care is essential to prevent pressure sores. Tilting beds may reduce the risk of pressure sores. Regular physiotherapy to limbs and the application of appropriate splints will limit the formation of contractures. All patients with a spinal cord injury should be referred to a specialist spinal injuries unit. If the patient cannot be transferred initially, the spinal injury specialist may be able to visit the patient and advise on management.

Crush injuries

Acute renal failure

Fluid and, if necessary, inotropes should be administered to restore cardiac output and renal perfusion. Intravenous bicarbonate may also be required to maintain the urine pH > 7.0, as alkalinisation will improve tubular washout of myoglobin and prevent lipid peroxidation and renal vasoconstriction. Mannitol has no advantage over volume expansion alone. If these measures fail to prevent acute renal failure, renal replacement therapy should be commenced early.

Compartment syndrome

Compartmental pressures should be measured, if a compartment syndrome is suspected. The normal technique is to use a transcutaneous needle or cannula, but this may introduce infection. Some clinicians advocate the use of indwelling intravascular catheters passed down into the relevant compartment. Fasciotomies are usually undertaken when compartment pressures exceed 40 mmHg.

Electrolyte complications

Hyperkalaemia should be corrected by volume expansion and an intravenous infusion of dextrose and insulin. The alkalinisation will not only improve myoglobin washout, but also help to reduce serum potassium levels. Intravenous calcium may cause heterotopic calcification in damaged muscle and should only be used for severe hyperkalaemia (i.e. >6.5 mmol.l^{-1}). If these measures fail to control hyperkalaemia, renal replacement therapy should be commenced early. This has the advantage of also correcting acidosis, hyperphosphataemia, hyperuricaemia and hypocalcaemia.

Long-term ventilation of spinal patients

Patients with a complete cord lesion above C4 will need long-term ventilation. As accessory muscle function improves, patients with C4/5 lesions may generate adequate alveolar ventilation to be independent of mechanical ventilation. Only 14–18% of patients with injuries below C5 require long-term assisted ventilation and this is usually because of pre-existing lung disease or mechanical dysfunction of the chest wall.

Portable ventilators can be mounted on a wheelchair to provide the patient with some independence and the use of an uncuffed tracheostomy tube will enable speech. Some patients are suitable for electrophrenic ventilation with an implanted phrenic nerve stimulator. If bulbar function is intact, non-invasive ventilation may be possible. Non-invasive assisted ventilation can be successful for patients with compromised respiratory function during the acute rehabilitation period as well as in the long term.

USUAL OUTCOMES

Spinal injuries

Effective resuscitation and careful spinal immobilisation has helped to reduce the proportion of complete spinal cord injuries from 50% to 39% of all patients with cord injuries. Hospital survival for spinal injury patients is now greater than 90% and over half of these achieve self-care and independence. Early transfer to a specialist spinal injury centre for intensive rehabilitation improves outcome.

Crush injuries

Twenty percent of patients who develop acute renal failure from rhabdomyolysis will die. Survivors will nearly always recover their renal function within 3 months.

KEY LEARNING POINTS

Spinal injuries

1. Prevention is better than treatment; all trauma patients should be managed as if they have a spinal injury until proven otherwise.

2. Careful attention to the airway, breathing and circulation will help prevent secondary cord injury.

3. Associated injuries are common and may be masked by the spinal injury; a high index of suspicion for both haemorrhagic and spinal shock is required.

4. Meticulous nursing care and physiotherapy is vital in helping to prevent long-term complications.

Crush injuries

1. Consider rhabdomyolysis and compartment syndrome in any patient with a history of crush injury, especially of the lower limbs.

2. Effective resuscitation is vital to avert acute renal failure, which has a high mortality in crush syndrome.

3. Watch for and treat electrolyte abnormalities.

Further reading

1. Cobby TF, Hardman JG, Baxendale BR. Anaesthetic management of the severely injured patient: spinal injury. *British Journal of Hospital Medicine* 1997; **58**: 198–201.

2. Wright SW, Robinson GG, Wright MB. Cervical spine injuries in blunt trauma patients requiring emergent endotracheal intubation. *American Journal of Emergency Medicine* 1992; **10**: 104–9.

3. Anderson DK, Hall ED. Pathophysiology of spinal cord trauma. *Annals of Emergency Medicine* 1993; **22**: 987–92.

4. Chiles BW, Cooper PR. Acute spinal injury. *New England Journal of Medicine* 1996; **334**: 514–20.

5. Boles JM. Rhabdomyolysis and compartment syndrome. In Webb AR, Shapiro MJ, Singer M, Suter PM (eds), *Oxford Textbook of Critical Care*. Oxford: Oxford University Press, 1999: 722–5.

6. Better OS, Stein JH. Early management of shock and prophylaxis of acute renal failure in traumatic rhabdomyolysis. *New England Journal of Medicine* 1990; **322**: 825–9.

7. Slater MS, Mullins RJ. Rhabdomyolysis and myoglobinuric renal failure in trauma and surgical patients: a review. *Journal of the American College of Surgeons* 1998; **186**: 693–716.

8. Holt SG, Moore KP. Pathogenesis and treatment of renal dysfunction in rhabdomyolysis. *Intensive Care Medicine* 2001; **27**: 803–11.

9. Grundy D, Swain A. *ABC of Spinal Cord Injury*, 3rd edn. London: BMJ Publishing Group, 1996.

10. McLeod ADM, Calder I. Spinal cord injury and direct laryngoscopy – the legend lives on. *British Journal of Anaesthesia* 2000; **84**: 705–8.

11. Bracken MB, Shepard MJ, Collins WF *et al*. Methylprednisolone or naloxone treatment after acute spinal cord injury: 1-year follow up data: results of the second National Acute Spinal Cord Injury Study. *Journal of Neurosurgery* 1992; **76**: 23–31.

12. Bracken MB, Shepard MJ, Holford TR *et al*. Administration of methylprednisolone for 24 or 48 hrs or tirilazad mesylate for 48 hours in the treatment of acute spinal cord injury. *Journal of the American Medical Association* 1997; **277**: 1597–604.

13. Viroslav J, Rosenblatt R, Tomazevic SM. Respiratory management, survival, and quality of life for high-level traumatic tetraplegics. *Respiratory Care Clinics of North America* 1996; **2**: 313–22.

14. Joynt GM, Young KK. Spinal injuries. In Oh TE (ed.), *Intensive Care Manual*. Oxford: Butterworth-Heinemann, 1997: 598–605.

20

MANAGEMENT OF AN OVERDOSE INVOLVING ALCOHOL AND UNKNOWN DRUGS

G B Smith

CASE SCENARIO

An 18-year-old female is admitted to hospital following a probable drug overdose. Her friends say that they found her in a confused state, some hours after a dispute with her boyfriend. Before lapsing into coma, she apparently told them she had taken '... *a large amount of alcohol and some drugs that belonged to her father* ...' He is being treated for depression. The patient is normally fit, active and healthy. When attended by the ambulance paramedics she had a Glasgow Coma Scale (GCS) score of 11, but this fell during transfer to hospital. The paramedics noticed that she was 'twitchy', had a tachycardia (125 beats.min^{-1}) and widely dilated pupils. On arrival at the Accident and Emergency (A&E) Department, she develops grand mal seizures. Her father cannot be contacted. No tablet containers were found at the scene. It is now approximately 2 hours since she took the presumed overdose.

DEFINITION AND DESCRIPTION OF THE PROBLEM

Poisoning accounts for approximately 2–3% of all urban A&E Department visits and leads to about 100 000 hospital admissions annually. It is a common cause of non-traumatic coma in patients aged below 35 years. The majority of poisonings involve medications, but occasionally inhalation of fumes or skin contact with a toxin is responsible. Poisoning may be intentional ($\approx$95%) or accidental; very occasionally, it results from malicious intention by a third party. There is often no clear history that allows confident identification of the poison or of the precise timing of exposure. Even in circumstances where this information is available or offered, it may be unreliable. Occasionally, especially where malice or the use of recreational drugs is involved, attempts may be made to conceal the true clinical history. In the UK, the most common acute poisonings are with tricyclic antidepressants (TCAs), salicylates, paracetamol, benzodiazepines, carbon monoxide and alcohol. About half of all poisonings involve a mixture of substances.

As is the case in many poisoning episodes, the patient described here has a reduced level of consciousness that places her at risk of airway obstruction, aspiration of vomit and damage to pressure areas. Many poisons also have both general and specific toxic effects on the respiratory, cardiac, circulatory, renal, thermoregulatory, neural and metabolic functions of the body. Poisoned patients may have pre-existing medical disease (e.g. coronary artery disease) such that the overdose is less well tolerated. Other patients may have illnesses that can influence the body's handling of a particular poison (e.g. renal failure).

Most poisoned patients, although often requiring hospital admission for observation, do not need intensive care unit (ICU) admission and are safely managed on general wards with little or no specific treatment. However, the development of life threatening complications, such as those described in the case history above, implies that ICU admission will be necessary.

PATHOLOGY AND PATHOPHYSIOLOGY OF POISONING AND OVERDOSE

Despite the wide range of agents that may be administered or taken in overdose, the signs and symptoms of poisoning often show remarkable similarity between agents (Table 20.1). This may make exact identification of the poison difficult, however, the recognition of specific 'toxidromes' – syndromes of signs and symptoms caused by groups of drugs (Table 20.2) – may make diagnosis easier.

Many agents cause a variable depression of conscious level that may lead to airway obstruction, depressed airway reflexes and reduced peripheral sensation and spontaneous motor activity. These make the patient prone to hypoxaemia and hypercapnia, aspiration of gastric contents and pressure area damage. Patients who remain unconscious for many hours before being found face the additional risks of hypothermia (due to depressed motor activity and metabolic rate), skin blistering, peripheral neuropathy and rhabdomyolysis. Central nervous system (CNS) depression also reduces the respiratory drive and may cause hypotension. Some agents, as well as being sedatives, are also central nervous stimulants and cause confusion (e.g. TCAs, amphetamines) or, more seriously, muscle spasm or convulsions (e.g. TCAs, carbon monoxide, theophylline).

Reduced ventilatory drive and reduced minute volume, resulting in a respiratory acidosis, are frequent effects of drugs responsible for poisoning. However, some

Table 20.1 – Common presenting symptoms in poisoning.

Sign	Possible causal agents
Bradycardia	Digoxin, β-adrenergic receptor antagonists, calcium-channel antagonists, organophosphates
Tachycardia	Cocaine, theophylline, TCAs, antihistamines
Hypertension	Monoamine oxidase inhibitors, cocaine, amphetamines
Hypotension	Barbiturates, opioids, digoxin, β-adrenergic receptor antagonists, calcium-channel antagonists
Tachypnoea and hyperventilation	Salicylates, methanol, ethylene glycol, carbon monoxide
Hypoventilation	Opioids, barbiturates, benzodiazepines, alcohol
Hypothermia	Barbiturates, ethanol, opioids, benzodiazepines
Hyperthermia	Phenothiazines, anticholinergic agents, salicylates, cocaine, ecstasy, monoamine oxidase inhibitors
Seizures	TCAs, theophylline
Cardiac dysrhythmias	TCAs, cocaine, anticholinergic agents
Mydriasis	Cocaine, TCAs, anticholinergic agents
Miosis	Organophosphates, opioids, clonidine
Breath odours	Alcohol, cyanide
Skin changes (colour, bullae)	Diffuse flushing (anticholinergics); cyanosis (methaemoglobinaemia); diaphoresis (sympathomimetics); cherry red skin (carbon monoxide); bullae (barbiturates)
Sedation	Opioids, benzodiazepines, barbiturates, TCAs, hypoglycaemic agents, cyanide, carbon monoxide
Agitation	Phencylcidine, TCAs, hypoglycaemic agents, sympathomimetic agents

Table 20.2 – Common 'toxidromes'.

Anticholinergic drugs, for example, antihistamines, atropine, TCAs, antispasmodics, antipsychotic agents	Tachycardia, dysrhythmias, delirium, coma, hyper-reflexia, myoclonus, seizures, dry skin, dilated pupils, urinary retention, ileus
Sympathomimetic agents, for example, amphetamines, ephedrine, caffeine, theophylline, cocaine	Delusions, paranoia, tachycardia, hypertension, diaphoresis, hyperthermia, mydriasis, hyper-reflexia
Opiates and sedatives, for example, barbiturates, benzodiazepines, opioids	Hyporeflexia, coma, miosis, respiratory depression, hypotension, bradycardia, hypothermia
Cholinergic, for example, organophosphate insecticides, edrophonium, some mushrooms	Confusion, CNS depression, bradycardia, muscle weakness, salivation, lacrimation, diaphoresis, urinary incontinence, muscle fasciculations

agents (e.g. salicylates) actually stimulate respiration, causing a respiratory alkalosis, while many others lead to a metabolic acidosis. Direct pulmonary damage may follow exposure to irritant gases or other agents such as paraquat.

The effect of poisons on the circulatory system is variable. Many agents depress the heart rate and/or myocardial contractility directly (e.g. beta-blockers, calcium antagonists) or cause severe tachydysrhythmias (e.g. TCAs) that interfere with contractility or precipitate cardiac arrest. Other agents have a predominant effect on the peripheral circulation (e.g. alpha-blockers). Conversely, taken in excess, amphetamines may cause tachycardia and severe life threatening hypertension by virtue of their sympathomimetic actions.

Some toxins are cellular poisons (e.g. cyanide, carbon monoxide, paracetamol); others (e.g. ecstasy, monoamine oxidase inhibitors) may cause hyperthermia that can lead to cellular damage. Cellular damage may be generalised (e.g. carbon monoxide, cyanide) or directed against specific tissues (e.g. paracetamol induced hepatic necrosis). Renal complications may result from hypotension or hypovolaemia, direct nephrotoxicity of the poison or rhabdomyolysis.

THERAPEUTIC GOALS

The therapeutic goals for this patient dictate that:

1. Efforts must be directed to addressing any deficiencies in the vital signs of the patient, with special emphasis on the patency of the airway (A), adequacy of breathing (B) and state of the circulation (C).

2. Where possible, the poison should be identified using a combination of circumstantial evidence, symptoms, clinical signs, results of blood investigations and abnormalities of acid–base disturbance. Information regarding the quantity ingested and time since ingestion should be gathered.

3. Attempts should be made to antagonise the effects of the poison, to limit the absorption of poison by the gastrointestinal tract (or other route, if appropriate), to accelerate its excretion by the body and to prevent the complications of overdose.

THERAPEUTIC OPTIONS BASED ON PHYSIOLOGICAL AND PHARMACOLOGICAL EFFECTS

Preventing and treating the immediate life threatening effects of poisoning

During the initial brief assessment of the patient, attention must be paid to ensuring that the ABCs (i.e. airway, breathing, circulation) are stabilised and that adequate oxygenation is achieved. At the same time, assessment of conscious level (e.g. using the AVPU scale or GCS) should be made, a blood sugar level measured and core body temperature obtained.

AVPU scale for assessing conscious level is:

-   **A** **A**lert
-   **V** Responds to **V**oice
-   **P** Responds to **P**ain
-   **U** **U**nresponsive

Abnormalities should be treated promptly. In the case under discussion, the main life threatening effect of the ingested agents is the development of grand mal seizures. Control of the airway, using rapid sequence induction of anaesthesia and intubation, and assisted ventilation may be required if seizure control is difficult or if the conscious level is severely depressed (i.e. GCS < 9). Where marked alterations in pH may result in changes in drug toxicity (e.g. TCAs) an attempt should be made to ensure that pH is controlled in such a way as to minimise exacerbating drug toxicity (e.g. ensure hyperventilation to promote alkalaemia in tricyclic poisoning).

Initially, seizure control following poisoning should be attempted using benzo-diazepines (diazemuls 2.5–10 mg boluses, followed by an infusion), but phenytoin (15 mg.kg^{-1} bolus, followed by an infusion) may also be required. If hypotension occurs, it should be treated along standard lines using intravenous fluids, and if necessary, using vasoactive drugs such as noradrenaline and dobutamine. If this is the case, central venous pressure monitoring should be used to guide therapy. The management of dysrhythmias requires careful consideration of the likely poison, as therapeutic drugs and poison may interact.

Poisoned patients require cardiorespiratory monitoring and frequent assessment of their neurological state. As protein binding, tissue levels, blood levels and the clinical effects of drugs may each be affected by acid–base changes, regular re-assessments are essential. It should be remembered that pulse oximetry has its limitations in poisoning, as it is not a monitor of ventilation and may be inaccurate in cases of carbon monoxide poisoning or where agents convert haemoglobin to methaemoglobin.

Identification of the drug or agent responsible for poisoning

It is often not possible to identify clearly the poison involved and circumstantial evidence must be used. Important clues can come from empty pill bottles, tablet markings and/or the spectrum of clinical signs (Tables 20.1 and 20.2). It should be remembered that patients may re-use tablet containers, filling them with unrelated drugs. Poisons are often taken in combination with alcohol and such mixtures tend to be synergistic. Urgent qualitative and quantitative laboratory analysis of blood may be helpful for some agents (e.g. salicylates and paracetamol) but is not immediately available for many others poisons, mainly because it rarely influences clinical management. Assistance in identifying agents may be gained from regional poisons centres, standard texts, or by later toxicological analysis of gastric aspirate, urine and blood. It should be remembered that not all poisons are taken orally; other clues may include injection marks and the existence of prior thrombophlebitis in intravenous drug abusers. Some drugs produce distinctive breath odours (e.g. alcohol, cyanide (burnt almonds)) that may assist in identification. In all cases of poisoning, it is essential to ensure that the clinical features are compatible with the assumed toxin. It is important to identify how much poison has been taken or administered and the time elapsed since exposure. Knowledge of the agent's pharmacodynamics and

Table 20.3 – Metabolic abnormalities due to poisoning.

Metabolic abnormality	Possible causal agents
Metabolic acidosis	Salicylate, methanol, ethylene glycol
Respiratory alkalosis	Salicylate
Respiratory acidosis	Opioids, benzodiazepines, barbiturates
Hypoglycaemia	Hypoglycaemia agents, insulin, alcohol
Methaemoglobinaemia	Amylnitrate, lead, nitroglycerin, prilocaine, sulphonamides
Increased anion gap	Salicylate, methanol, ethylene glycol
Increased osmolar gap	Ethanol, methanol, ethylene glycol

pharmacokinetics (e.g. slow release preparations) is important, as it may affect the therapeutic options. Occasionally, serum biochemistry results will give a clue (e.g. metabolic acidosis in salicylate, alcohol, cyanide poisoning; increased osmolal gap in alcohol poisoning and increased anion gap in salicylate poisoning) (Table 20.3). The electrocardiogram (ECG) may also assist in diagnosis.

Analysis of the available history, symptoms and signs in the case history described above suggests that this patient's overdose is a combination of alcohol and TCA drugs. TCAs are most often used for the treatment of endogenous depression, although they are also used in the treatment of panic attacks and some forms of neuralgia. Commonly prescribed agents include amitryptyline, imipramine, dothiepin, doxepin, lofepramine and amoxapine. TCAs have marked anticholinergic side effects that result in a series of symptoms and signs, many of which are not life threatening. The potentially lethal effects of these drugs are due to their actions on the cardiovascular and CNS. TCA overdose causes about 250 deaths each year in the UK.

TCAs affect the cardiovascular system by three mechanisms. Firstly, their anticholinergic effects cause a sinus tachycardia and mildly increased blood pressure. Secondly, TCAs block the uptake of noradrenaline at adrenergic pre-synaptic endings, thereby causing noradrenaline to accumulate in the synapse. This leads to increased stimulation of both central and peripheral adrenergic neurons, resulting in tachycardia, hypertension and an elevated cardiac output. Eventually, myocardial depression and hypotension result from noradrenaline depletion. Finally, TCAs have a membrane stabilising effect that depresses the excitability of nerve and muscle cells. This leads to an increased refractory period, raised stimulation threshold and decreased automaticity of cardiac muscle cells. The resulting electrophysiological effects are manifest on ECG by prolonged PR interval, prolonged QRS complexes (often with bizarre morphology), prolonged QT_c interval (i.e. QT interval corrected for ventricular rate), ventricular extrasystoles, ventricular tachycardia and ventricular fibrillation (Figure 20.1). Eventually, profound bradycardia with variable atrioventricular block may occur. Although TCAs are thought to have an α-adrenergic receptor blocking action, this does not seem to be responsible for hypotension in cases of TCA overdose.

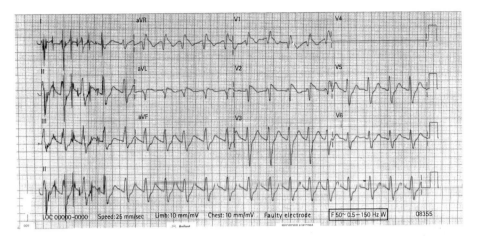

Figure 20.1 – ECG with long QT$_c$ and wide QRS. The ECG of a patient following a TCA overdose. Note several features: the QRS complexes are wide, the QT$_c$ is prolonged (−0.66 s), there is evidence of seizure activity in leads I, II and III; lead V4 has fallen off during the seizure. Normal range for QT$_c$ is 0.35–0.43 s. The QT$_c$ is calculated using Bazet's formula: QT$_c$ = QT internal/$\sqrt{(R-R \text{ internal})}$.

Although the central anticholinergic actions of excess TCAs may cause agitation, delirium, ataxia or hallucinations, many patients will present in coma. This usually starts within 6 h of ingestion and, on average, lasts approximately 24 h. Its onset may be very rapid and underlines the need for constant observation of TCA overdose victims in hospital. Of more concern is the tendency of TCAs in overdose to cause twitching, myoclonic jerking and grand mal seizures. Depending on the TCA ingested, seizures may result from alterations in serotoninergic, dopaminergic, noradrenergic and cholinergic systems. Other signs of toxicity include hyper-reflexia and extensor plantar responses. In severe poisoning, reversible loss of brain stem reflexes is possible. Other signs and symptoms of TCA poisoning include dry mouth, urinary retention, dilated pupils, ileus and gastroparesis.

In normal therapeutic doses, TCAs are absorbed within 2 h. However, in overdose, their absorption is slowed because the drug is ionised in the acid conditions of the stomach and the drug inhibits peristalsis and causes gastric dilatation. The distribution of TCAs within the body depends to a major extent on the degree of ionisation of the drug. Low pH favours ionisation of the drug, which decreases lipid solubility of the drug. Plasma binding is decreased by a low pH. Blood levels of TCAs following overdose cannot be used consistently and reliably for determining treatment or prognosis, predominantly because the amount of TCA in plasma is usually small in comparison with that in tissues. Additionally, TCA levels can fluctuate rapidly and the assays may be unreliable; some TCA metabolites are more toxic than their parent drug.

From the history, it seems that this patient took the poisons in conjunction with alcohol. The most common pattern following the ingestion of excess alcohol is a lack of inhibition, slurred speech, non-coordination, sensory loss, sedation, coma, flaccidity, convulsions, vasodilatation, and hypotension. Hypoglycaemia, due to inhibition of gluconeogenesis, and, rarely, metabolic acidosis may also occur.

Use of antidotes

Some of the commonly taken poisons have antidotes that can reverse the effects of the poison and minimise side effects (Table 20.4). In general, these act by competitive antagonism, immunological binding, chelation or affecting metabolic pathways. In many A&E Departments, the most commonly used competitive antagonists, naloxone and flumazenil, are often administered empirically without danger. However, the reversal of benzodiazepine-induced sedation with flumazenil is dangerous if undertaken in a patient poisoned with a combination of benzodiazepines and TCAs, as it will often provoke seizures. Flumazenil and naloxone have shorter half-lives than the agonist drugs they reverse. Consequently, infusions of these drugs may be required to maintain consciousness.

Currently, only a few drugs (notably digoxin) can be reversed by specific antibody complexes, although it is likely that TCA poisoning may be managed in this way in the near future. Many heavy metals may be bound by chelating agents that incorporate the metal ions within the inner ring structure of the chelating molecule. The toxic effects of other drugs are minimised by antidotes that act via the drug's metabolic pathways. For instance, paracetamol taken in excess may cause severe hepatocellular necrosis or acute tubular necrosis. The metabolite of paracetamol,

Table 20.4 – Specific antidotes to poisons.

Antidote	Poison
Calcium chloride	Calcium channel blocking agents
Cobalt edetate	Lead, cyanide
Desferrioxamine	Iron
Digibind	Digoxin
Ethanol	Methanol, ethylene glycol
Flumazenil	Benzodiazepines
Fuller's earth	Paraquat
Glucagon	β-Adrenergic receptor antagonists
Methylene blue	Methaemoglobinaemia
Naloxone	Opiates
N-acetylcysteine	Paracetamol
Oxygen	Carbon monoxide
Pralidoxime	Organophosphates
Sodium thiosulphate	Cyanide
Vitamin K	Warfarin

n-acetyl-p-benzoquinoneimine, is usually detoxified by liver glutathione; however, the normal stores of this are small and are soon depleted if excess n-acetyl-p-benzoquinoneimine is presented to the liver. An intravenous antidote, n-actylcysteine, administered according to a treatment nomogram will replenish depleted glutathione stores thereby preventing toxicity.

Although not truly an antidote, the use of intravenous sodium bicarbonate $(1–2\,mmol.kg^{-1}$ body weight) to produce alkalaemia appears to reduce the risk of dysrhythmias, and possibly seizures, in TCA poisoning. However, at present, its efficacy, the optimal dose and administration rate (i.e. bolus versus infusion) have not been established. It is also possible that hyperventilation may be as effective. There is currently no agreed end-point to therapy and the issue of whether bicarbonate treatment should be reactive or prophylactic is unresolved. However, a pragmatic approach may be needed to ensure that the patient has a neutral pH or alkalaemia or to start sodium bicarbonate therapy, if the QRS interval is prolonged (i.e. $>0.14\,s$).

Limiting of absorption

Limiting absorption of agents from the gut may be achieved by either removing the drug from the stomach, preventing the uptake of ingested drug or shortening the transit time of the drug through the gastrointestinal system.

Removal of the agent from the stomach

Emesis

In the past, removal of ingested poison was undertaken using a method that would induce emesis. The most commonly used pharmacological agent was ipecacuanha syrup (a mixture of two plant alkaloids, emetine and cephaeline) that induces emesis by direct gastric mucosal irritation and stimulation of the chemoreceptor trigger zone. As the use of ipecacuanha delays the administration or reduces the efficacy of activated charcoal, oral antidotes or whole bowel irrigation, it is no longer employed on a routine basis. There is no evidence that it prevents clinically significant absorption of drugs and should only be considered in fully conscious patients where the poison is not absorbed by activated charcoal (see below) or if gastric lavage is inadvisable or refused. It should not be used if the patient has a reduced conscious level.

Gastric lavage

Direct removal of an ingested poison using simple gastric lavage has doubtful benefits unless it can be undertaken within 60 min of the poison's ingestion. One significant exception to this rule may be, when significant amounts of salicylates have been ingested, as they will slow peristaltic activity in the stomach and may be recoverable for many hours afterwards. Lavage is associated with significant morbidity, especially pulmonary aspiration, and should not be used in patients with a reduced conscious level or if the agent is corrosive or petroleum based.

Limitation of absorption of the poison

The use of a single dose of 50 g of activated charcoal to bind poison in the stomach may be considered if the patient has ingested a potentially toxic amount of a poison up to 1h previously. It is particularly effective in the management of poisoning with agents that are toxic in small amounts (e.g. antidepressants). However, charcoal is not effective against all agents, becoming less effective with time, and should only be used if the patient's airway is protected. The use of multiple doses of activated charcoal (usually 50 g 4 hourly) has advantages over other 'blood purification' techniques as it is less invasive. However, it may cause constipation or even bowel obstruction with a charcoal stercolith and there is a risk of pulmonary aspiration of charcoal. Repeated administration of activated charcoal is thought to act by three mechanisms (intraluminal adsorption, interrupting the enterohepatic circulation of drugs and 'intestinal dialysis'). If used, repeated use of charcoal should probably be reserved for patients with known ingestion of life threatening amounts of carbemazepine, phenytoin, salicylate, phenobarbital, quinine or theophylline.

Removal of toxin from the gastrointestinal tract

Cathartics

Cathartics such as magnesium sulphate or hydroxide are used to stimulate bowel activity by drawing water into the gastrointestinal tract by osmosis, thereby encouraging expulsion of the toxin. Although intuitive, there is little evidence that this results in reduced toxin absorption. Adverse effects of this technique, including dehydration and electrolyte abnormalities, imply that it has a limited role, especially, at extremes of age.

Whole bowel irrigation

This technique has become increasingly popular, particularly for overdoses of sustained release or enteric-coated poisons. It may also have a role if drugs are ingested in drug-filled packets or if activated charcoal is ineffective for the agent concerned (e.g. iron, lithium, lead). Whole bowel irrigation involves the use of large volumes of isosmolar, isotonic, non-absorbable bowel cleansing solutions, containing polyethylene glycol and electrolytes, to produce copious amounts of liquid stool. The technique is contraindicated if there is bowel obstruction, perforation, ileus or haemodynamic instability.

Active removal of poison from the circulation and body tissues

Once poisons have been absorbed, techniques are required that will accelerate their removal from the circulation and tissues. Although repeated doses of activated charcoal may assist, other methods exist.

Forced diuresis and urinary pH manipulation

Encouraging diuresis by using intravenous infusion fluid alone, or combining it with frusemide or dopamine, will accelerate the amount of poison removed per minute. Usually, forced diuresis is combined with urinary pH manipulation, taking advantage of the alteration in ionisation of drugs that are variably ionised according to environmental pH. For instance, the generation of alkaline urine by administering intravenous sodium bicarbonate will increase the degree of ionisation of salicylate within the renal tubular lumen, thereby enhancing its elimination. Similarly, the use of ammonium chloride to produce acid urine will increase the degree of ionisation of drugs such as amphetamines and result in greater amounts excreted. If forced diuresis methods are used, it is important to monitor fluid balance closely and to be aware that pulmonary or cerebral oedema are possible complications.

Haemodialysis and haemoperfusion

These techniques are usually reserved for situations in which simpler, less-invasive methods have failed. The complications from both haemodialysis and haemoperfusion are potentially serious as systemic anticoagulation, an extracorporeal circuit and large vein cannulation are required. Air embolism is also a potential risk. Neither technique is useful for agents with high tissue binding. Haemodialysis is most useful for agents that are highly soluble in water, have low protein binding and a low molecular weight (e.g. alcohol, salicylate, lithium), whereas haemoperfusion is better, if the drug is poorly water soluble or highly protein bound (e.g. theophylline).

Haemofiltration and haemodiafiltration

These techniques are not as effective as haemodialysis or haemoperfusion in the management of acute poisoning, as the clearance of drugs or toxins is considerably less.

In the case of combined TCA and alcohol poisoning described, treatment is mainly supportive and none of the methods described for limiting the absorption of agents from the gut or increasing the rate of removal from the body are, particularly, useful.

USUAL OUTCOME

The majority of poisoned patients will recover fully with supportive therapy, use of antidotes and attention to correct management of complications of the toxins, such as seizures and dysrhythmias. Few, except those with severe poisoning or with marked cardiovascular, respiratory or neurological complications, require admission to an ICU. Although secondary complications such as deep venous thrombosis, pulmonary embolism, gastrointestinal haemorrhage and pneumonia do occur, they are uncommon. Consequently, the outcome from poisoning is usually extremely good, but will obviously depend upon the agent involved. ICU mortality is approximately 1–2%. Patients admitted to hospital after overdose require careful psychiatric assessment with regard to the likelihood of further self-harm, including suicide.

KEY LEARNING POINTS

1. Common presenting features in poisoning include depressed consciousness, airway obstruction, hypoventilation, hypotension, dysrhythmias, cardiorespiratory arrest, seizures and hypothermia.

2. Most poisoned patients can be managed using simple attention to the airway, breathing and circulation.

3. Emesis and gastric lavage have very limited roles in the current practice of managing poisoned patients. However, the use of activated charcoal, cathartic agents or whole bowel irrigation may be used to remove toxins from the gastrointestinal tract.

4. A range of specific antidotes may be useful in reducing or reversing the effects of poisons.

5. Forced diuresis, urinary pH manipulation, haemodialysis and haemoperfusion may have a place in the management of specific poisons. However, haemofiltration and haemodiafiltration are not, particularly, effective.

6. The outcome from poisoning is usually extremely good, but will obviously depend upon the agent involved. ICU mortality is approximately 1–2%.

Further reading

1. Manoguerra AS. Gastrointestinal decontamination after poisoning: where is the science? *Critical Care Clinics* 1997; **4**: 709–25.

2. Henderson A, Wright M, Pond SM. Experience with 732 acute overdose patients admitted to an intensive care unit over six years. *Medical Journal of Australia* 1993; **158**: 28–30.

3. Vernon DD, Gleich MC. Poisoning and drug overdose. *Critical Care Clinics* 1997; **3**: 647–67.

4. Henry J, Volans G. *ABC of Poisoning*. London: British Medical Association, 1984.

5. Anonymous. Advanced challenges in resuscitation. Section 2: Toxicology in ECC. *Resuscitation* 2000; **46**: 261–6.

INDEX